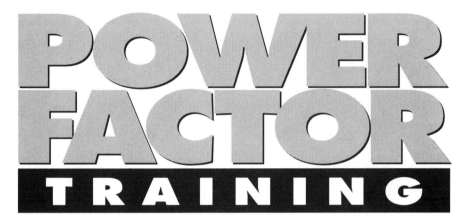

POWER FACTOR
TRAINING

A Scientific Approach to Building Lean Muscle Mass

PETER SISCO AND JOHN LITTLE

D0067481

CB
CONTEMPORARY BOOKS

Library of Congress Cataloging-in-Publication Data

Sisco, Peter.
    Power factor training : a scientific approach to building lean muscle
mass / Peter Sisco and John Little.
        p.   cm.
    Includes index.
    ISBN 0-8092-3071-2
    1. Bodybuilding—Physiological aspects.   I. Little, John.   II. Title.
RC1220.W44S57   1997
613.7'11—dc21   97-2345
                                            CIP

Cover design by Todd Petersen
Cover photo and interior photos by Mitsuru Okabe
Interior design by Hespenheide Design

Published by Contemporary Books
A division of NTC/Contemporary Publishing Group, Inc.
4255 West Touhy Avenue, Lincolnwood (Chicago), Illinois 60712-1975 U.S.A.
Printed in the United States of America
International Standard Book Number: 0-8092-3071-2

00 01 02 03 04 05 ML 20 19 18 17 16 15 14 13 12 11 10 9 8 7 6 5

This book is dedicated to every bodybuilder and athlete who has an inquiring, rational mind; to every person who can throw off the chains of comfortable habit and unproven premises and move in a new direction that is guided by reason and observational evidence, no matter where that direction takes him; to every person who tries a thing and immediately thinks, "How can I make this better?"; to every person who is unafraid to challenge the false beliefs of the herd and lead others out of the caves and into the light.

In the parlance of bodybuilding, it is the people with these "genes" who are truly the greatest champions of the human race. To these people, not just in the science of human strength but in every science, we owe our enormous gratitude.

CAUTION: This program involves a systematic progression of muscular overload that leads to the lifting of extremely heavy weights. As a result, a proper warm-up of muscles, tendons, ligaments, and joints is mandatory at the beginning of every workout.

WARNING: As this is a very intense program, it requires both a thorough knowledge of proper exercise form and a base level of strength fitness. Although exercise is very beneficial, the potential for injury does exist, especially if the trainee is not in good physical condition. Always consult with your physician before beginning any program of progressive weight training or exercise. If you feel any strain or pain when you are exercising, stop immediately and consult your physician.

Contents

Foreword

Arthur Jones once said to a young Mike Mentzer, "Muscles aren't the measure of a man." Since man's mind is his biologically distinctive trait, his means of survival, which can only be used by a volitional effort, an act of choice, the degree of its development in an individual is the proper standard by which to evaluate him.

John Little has never won a physique title, but he has been a serious bodybuilder for over fifteen years. More important is the fact that, unlike most bodybuilders (including the top champions), John has exerted considerable effort over a long period of time studying the actual science of productive bodybuilding exercise. He has acquired a firm intellectual understanding of the theory of high-intensity training.

Within the framework of that theory, John and Power Factor Training codeveloper Peter Sisco have developed a unique application that emphasizes very heavy overloading of the musculature using partial rep training. Taking into account the magnitude of the toll that such effort exacts on the body's limited recovery ability, they advocate much longer rest periods between workouts than most high-intensity training theorists.

Not only is their Power Factor Training theoretically sound, they have solid evidence that it works. Over the many months that John and Peter used and developed Power Factor Training, John reported to me periodically the fabulous results they were achieving.

For those seeking not only better results, but also a better understanding of the science of productive bodybuilding exercise, you have in your possession a book of enormous value.

MIKE MENTZER, MR. UNIVERSE

Definitions

"First, let us define our terms."—Socrates

SETS, REPS, and POWER FACTORS: The Jargon of Power Factor Training

Individuals who engage in bodybuilding are a genuine subculture of the population. Consequently, the practitioners of this sport use a jargon that, to outsiders, sounds as foreign as Caesar's Latin. Terms such as *reps, bi's, tri's, supersets, pre-exhaustion, forced reps,* and *negatives* are common to the bodybuilder but leave the initiate looking like a deer caught in the headlights of an oncoming car.

The terms of the bodybuilder, fortunately, are not as intimidating as they may at first appear. Further, it's not even necessary for the average athlete to learn more than a quarter of them. Many terms relate to advanced techniques of training, so they are not necessary for the purposes of 99 percent of trainees. We will concentrate on the few that you need to know in order to understand Power Factor Training.

REP: Shorthand for a repetition: the contraction and/or extension of a muscle group from a starting position of full extension to a finish position of full contraction and its subsequent return to the starting position. A series of such movements is, naturally enough, described as repetitions (reps).

SETS: A collection of repetitions (anywhere from one to one hundred or more). Generally, a brief rest of thirty to ninety seconds is taken after performing a series of repetitions. The rest between sets allows the trainee to catch his breath and provides time for the muscle group involved in the set to partially recuperate.

POUNDAGE: The amount of weight or resistance used on an exercise.

ONE-REP MAXIMUM: The heaviest amount of resistance that you can lift for one repetition.

ROUTINE: The sum of reps, sets, and exercises in any given workout or training session.

OVERLOAD (muscular overload): The total amount of work performed by the muscles while lifting weights.

PROGRESSIVE OVERLOAD: An increasing progression, from workout to workout, of the total amount of work performed by the muscles while lifting weights. Only when the overload reaches an amount greater than what the muscles are normally used to performing does an adaptive response (growth) take place.

POWER FACTOR (PF): A measurement of the intensity of muscular overload during an exercise. The Power Factor is measured in pounds per minute: $PF = \frac{W}{t}$, where *PF* is the Power Factor, *W* is the total weight lifted in pounds, and *t* is the total time in minutes.

POWER INDEX (P_i): A measurement of the duration of a given Power Factor. It is expressed as $P_i = \frac{W^2}{t} \times 10^{-6}$, where P_i is the Power Index, *W* is the total weight lifted, and *t* is the total time in minutes. The Power Index is measured on a logarithmic scale and is intended as a relative indicator of muscular output. There are no units of measurement. The Power Factor and Power Index measurements are innovations of Peter N. Sisco.

PRODUCTIVE WORKOUT: A workout of sufficient overload to trigger a growth response in the central nervous system, causing an increase in muscle size and strength.

A BRIEF LESSON IN ANATOMY AND PHYSIOLOGY

Before you can effectively train your muscles, you need to know how they function so you can select the exercises best suited to stimulate them to grow. Without making this a complicated physiological dissertation, let's examine just a few of our bodies' basic structures, the way they work together, and how this knowledge will make you more successful in your quest to build a stronger and better-looking body.

CENTRAL NERVOUS SYSTEM (CNS): The spinal cord and brain. The CNS functions in conjunction with the peripheral nervous system, which consists of the ganglia and nerves that reside outside of the brain and spinal cord. The nervous system appears like thousands of little wires that function as transmitters, receivers, and interpreters of data from all parts of the body. It is responsible for stimulating the muscles of your body to contract. It is of vital importance to both the aspiring and competitive bodybuilder as, without nerves, we'd be immobilized because our muscles wouldn't contract.

LIGAMENTS: Fibrous bands that bind bone to bone. Their compactness determines to a very large extent the flexibility of the joints they serve. Caution must be exercised when training because, if a ligament is stretched too far, the joint it holds together will become loose, resulting in permanent damage to this tissue.

TENDONS: Dense bands at the ends of muscles. Their function is to attach muscle to bone. In the tendons themselves are the Golgi tendon organs, which send signals to the brain indicating stress and fatigue levels. Generally, the ache that you experience during strenuous exercise is being transmitted via the tendon, not the muscle.

BONES: The hard connective tissue that makes up the skeleton. The human skeleton consists of 206 bones. Bones move when pulled by muscles attached to bones by tendons.

MUSCLES: Body tissue that can contract and produce motion. The body has three distinct kinds of muscle tissue: cardiac, smooth, and skeletal. Cardiac muscle is in the heart. Smooth muscle assists organs such as the stomach and intestines in the passage and digestion of food. Skeletal muscles are responsible for moving our bones. Power Factor Training increases the size of the skeletal muscles. The human body has over 600 skeletal muscles—a ratio of almost three skeletal muscles to every bone, which accounts for our highly evolved dexterity and precision in movement.

HYPERTROPHY: The process of increasing muscle size. The process itself isn't as complicated as some authors may have led you to believe. It occurs as a direct result of demands placed upon a muscle and the nervous system that is attached to it. The signal for hypertrophy is overload, that is, making the muscle work harder than it is normally accustomed to. To overload a muscle, you need to apply a load or a resistance for the muscle to contract against, and that resistance must be progressive from one workout to the next.

That's it. The bottom line in the quest for bigger and stronger muscles is progressive resistance. If you're able to increase your resistance by your next workout, it's because your muscles have overcompensated from your previous training session by getting bigger and stronger.

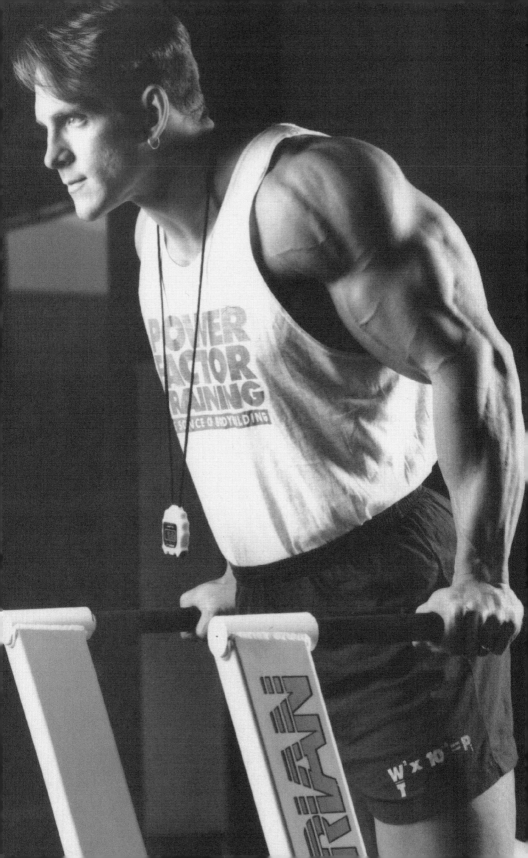

Understanding the Fundamentals

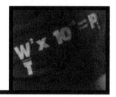

As this printing of *Power Factor Training* goes to press, at least twenty thousand athletes and body-builders in fifty-eight countries are training with this system and achieving their best results ever. What exactly is Power Factor Training? How did it originate? And why is it so effective?

To provide answers to these questions, we must begin by explaining the very nature of the muscle growth process. To begin with, muscle growth is a product of hypertrophy, or the enlarging of existing muscle cells. This was established about a hundred years ago by the research of Morpurgo and has been reaffirmed conclusively ever since.[1] The process of hypertrophy is one of muscular adaptation to imposed overload and occurs only through an increase in the cross-sectional area of a muscle's fibers. The task of causing muscle to grow can only be triggered by overloading a muscle. That's why we lift weights.

Power Factor Training provides you with a means to measure the effectiveness of any individual exercise.

Power Factor Training will provide you with a simple method to quantify the amount of muscular overload that you generate with every exercise and every workout. It will provide you with a means to measure the effectiveness of any individual exercise. Perhaps most important, it will provide a means to completely avoid overtraining and to ensure that every workout is productive. That degree of precision is unheard of in bodybuilding. In the past, trainees just adopted a training method that sounded good, followed it for several weeks or months, then attempted to subjectively assess whether it had worked. Most methods did not.

Power Factor Training works in 100 percent of cases because it strictly obeys the two fundamentals of muscle growth: high intensity of muscular overload and progressive overload. It obeys these in every exercise and in every workout. In any human of normal, healthy physiology, regardless of age or gender, following these two fundamentals will lead to bigger, stronger muscles.

THE OVERLOAD EQUATION

The term *overload* has come to be regarded as synonymous with the amount of weight a muscle is made to contract against; the heavier the weight, the greater the muscular overload. However, as far back as 1956, it was demonstrated clinically that weight per se is only part (although a large part admittedly) of the hypertrophy equation.[2]

The other indispensable element in the muscle growth process is the amount of work your muscles are made to perform in a given unit of time, which is measured in pounds per minute. Properly defined, maximum overload is the greatest possible muscular output over a given unit of time. Research conducted by Roux-Lange indicated, "Only when a muscle performs with greatest power, i.e., through the overcoming of a greater resistance in a unit of time than before, will its functional cross section need to increase. . . . Hypertrophy is seen only in muscles that must perform a great amount of work in a unit of time."[3] Further research by Petow and Siebert put a finer point on the issue of overload (intensity/ duration): "Hypertrophy results from an increase in the intensity of work done (increase of work in a unit time), whereas the total amount of work done is without significance."[4]

These results are significant for a number of reasons, particularly for "clean" athletes (natural trainees). First, they were obtained a full ten years before testosterone was first isolated, so all of the subjects participating in the study were unquestionably "natural," that is, of normal human endocrinology. Today, in contrast, drug testing of experimental subjects represents a prohibitive and impractical cost, so not all conclusions obtained from current training research can be said to apply to natural bodybuilders. Further, the research conclusions just quoted demonstrate clinically that, for clean athletes, the volume of muscular output (pounds per minute) is the sole contributing factor to the process of muscle growth. Additional research conducted by Dr. Arthur H. Steinhaus indicates, "Only when intensity is increased [overload] does hypertrophy follow."[5]

The implications of such data are certainly startling in light of many current training trends. For instance, in the context of these results, the belief that natural bodybuilders need periodization (for example, factoring into your workout schedule periods of lower muscular output) to stimulate muscle growth doesn't ring true. In fact, these studies prove conclusively that muscle grows larger solely in proportion to the pounds per minute work volume (the overload) applied to it. The greater the intensity or overload, the greater the hypertrophy.

Think about this for a moment. Once overload has been clearly isolated as the sole stimulus that induces muscular hypertrophy, then it logically follows that a training method that provides the greatest overload will stimulate the greatest muscle growth. It was this unambiguous conclusion that led to the development of Power Factor Training.

THE POWER FACTOR

Using Power Factor Training, you will be able to calculate a precise Power Factor and Power Index for each exercise you perform and for your entire workout. You will also be able to calculate ahead of time what workout you will be required to perform next time out in order to meet your goals of increased size and strength. This means that every workout can pay off in gains; if it doesn't, you'll know exactly where and why you fell short. You may, for example, find that your shrug power went down 7 percent even when your bench press power went up 34 percent and your overall Power Index went up 200 points. This level of precision and isolation truly represents a revolution in strength training.

MAXIMIZING MUSCULAR OVERLOAD

While the computations used in Power Factor Training can measure the muscular output of any exercise or training method, we quickly discovered that one method combined with specific exercises yielded the highest muscular output and, hence, the highest level of muscle growth stimulation. That method was partial repetitions performed in the muscle's strongest range of motion.

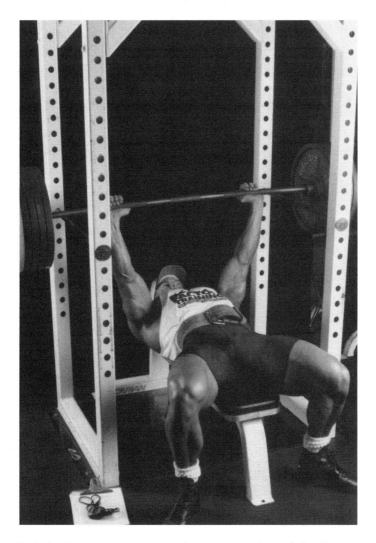

In the bench press, strongest range of motion occurs during the last few inches of your reach.

Using the bench press as an example, the weakest range of motion is where you first move the weight up a few inches from your chest. The strongest range, however, occurs during the last few inches of your reach. Training in the strongest range of motion allows you to employ tremendously heavy weights. The heavier the weights employed, the greater the muscular output and, of course, the resulting hypertrophy.

We once supervised the workouts of a subject whose maximum workout weight on the bench press was 200 pounds. He was limited to this weight because that was the most he could handle while training in his weakest range. However, we quickly discerned that his muscles were capable of handling much more resistance than he had been providing them; he was, in fact, capable of using 365 pounds for repetitions in his strongest range. But because he was locked into the notion that he had to perform full-range reps ("to develop the full muscle"), only the amount of fibers required to move 200 pounds were ever called into play. Once he started training with the maximum weight that his muscles were capable of lifting in his strongest range, his size and strength grew consistently. The contention that he required a full range of motion in order to build the entire breadth and length of his muscles has been proven erroneous owing to innervation, the fiber recruitment process, and the nature of overload training.

All academics aside, it simply stands to reason that training to failure in your strongest range of motion with much heavier weights is a lot more intense and demanding than training to failure in your weakest range of motion. Since the weights are heavier, more muscle fibers are required and activated to move them. Further, the recovery period following such a workout must also be greater. Why? Simply because the greater weights, combined with the greater muscular output required to move them, results in a greater depth of systemic fatigue.

THE THREE PHASES OF MUSCLE GROWTH

For muscular mass to increase, three distinct phases must take place. First, growth must be stimulated within the body. As we've learned, this can only be accomplished through subjecting your muscles (and, more specifically, your nervous system)[6] to a high level of muscular output, or what Roux-Lange called "a great amount of work in a unit of time."

The second phase is that of recovery. Both the body and the systems that feed the body must be given time to clean up the metabolic waste products of the workout and to replenish their energy reserves after a very draining maximum-overload workout. In fact, we've recently learned that completing this process can take anywhere from two or three days to six weeks or more, depending upon the level of muscular output employed during the training session and the subject's innate adaptability to exercise.

The third and final phase is the growth process itself, which will take place only after the recovery process has run its course. At least one study indicated that the actual growth of muscle may occur in as little as fifteen minutes during sleep. However, you must remember that in no case will muscle growth occur until adequate stimulation has been achieved and total recovery is complete. There is no way to force your body to skip steps one and two. It's always stimulate, recover, grow. Stimulate, recover, grow.

LOCALIZED MUSCLE RECOVERY VS. SYSTEMIC RECOVERY

With Power Factor Training, it's been established that working out even as little as three days per week can quickly lead to overtraining. This does not refer simply

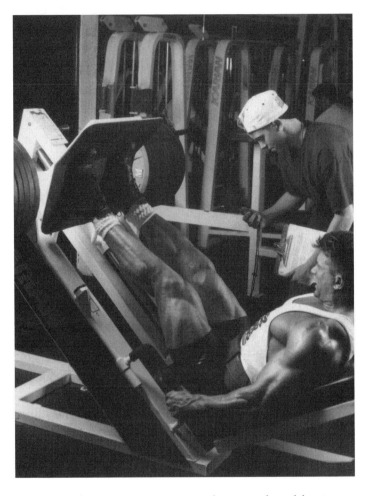

Training to failure in your strongest range of motion with much heavier weights is a lot more intense and demanding than training to failure in your weakest range of motion.

to localized muscle recovery but rather to the recovery of the physical system as a whole. Localized muscular recovery actually takes place very rapidly (in twenty-four hours in some cases). If you perform 10 sets of heavy squats on Monday, your legs may well have recovered by Tuesday. But try to do a heavy back workout! You won't feel the inclination. The reason is simply that your whole system is called upon whenever you exercise. When you trained your legs the day before, demands were made upon all of your body's recuperative subsystems (kidneys, liver, pancreas, etc.), not just your legs.

Since your whole system is called upon every time you work out, you've got to allow the whole system time to recover after each workout—not just the specific body part that you trained. This fact gave rise to Sisco's maxim: "Every day is kidney day."

SPECIFICITY OF TRAINING

Specific training methods result in specific training effects. In physiology circles, this is known as the specific adaptation to imposed demands (SAID) principle and is among the most fundamental to a proper understanding of the cause-and-effect relationship between exercise and muscle growth. We'll say more about this important physiological principle later in this book. For now, suffice it to say that when you train specifically for size and strength (training in your strongest range of motion with maximum overload), the results will come rapidly in proportion to the overload you impose on your muscles and their corresponding output. Conversely, if you train nonspecifically (that is, with full-range movements), the neuromuscular training stimulus is divided at least two different ways: (1) muscular size and strength and (2) flexibility. As a result, flexibility may be increased but at the expense of maximum muscular development. Exercising in the strongest range of motion, using partials, ignores the development of flexibility in favor of maximizing muscular overload.

Full range of motion is not a requirement for overloading a muscle, and overload is the only systemic stimulus that results in muscle growth. Granted, some overload is provided by full-range movements, but that overload is not anywhere near what it has the potential to be, as evidenced by the reduced poundages you're restricted to utilizing. Admittedly, some individuals such as Bill Kazmaier, Dorian Yates, and Flex Wheeler can use some phenomenal poundages for full-range reps, but this only goes to show that the weak range of motion for these particular trainees is tremendously strong—certainly much stronger than for the average trainee. However, if their weak range of motion is this strong, their strongest range of motion by definition would be even greater. Hence, it is capable of recruiting and stimulating even more muscle fibers, thereby increasing their muscle growth potential.

NOTES

1. Morpurgo, Ueber Activitats-hypertrophle der wikurlichen Muskein, *Virchows Arch.*, 150, 522–44 (1897). Morpurgo's research was corroborated by the experiments of physiologists such as W. Siebert & H. Petow, Studien uber Arbeitshypertrophie des Muskels, Z. Klin Med, 102, 427–33 (1925), and Untersuchungen uber Hypoertrophie des Skellet-muskels, Z. Klin Med, 109, 350–59 (1928); Leeberger, Professor of Physical Education, University of California (who presented his findings at an annual meeting of the American Association of Health, Physical Education and Recreation [AAHPER] in 1932); Barnett, Holly & Ashmore, Stretch-induced growth in chicken wing muscles: biochemical and morphological characterization, *Am. J. of Phys.*, 239, C39–46 (1980); Atherton, James & Mahon, Studies on muscle fiber splitting in skeletal muscle, *Experientia*, 37, 308–10 (1981); and Gollnick, Timson, Moore & Reidy, Muscular enlargement and number of fibers in skeletal muscles of rats, *J. App. Phys.*, 50, 936–43 (1981), to name but a few.

2. F. A. Hellebrandt & S. J. Houtz, *Physical Therapy Review*, 36 (1956).

3. Roux-Lange, *Usher Funktionelle Anpassung USW* (Berlin: Julius Springer, 1917).

4. W. Siebert & H. Petow, Studien uber Arbeitshypertrophie des Muskels.

5. A. Steinhaus, Strength from Morpurgo to Miller—a half century of research, *J. Assn. Physical & Mental Rehab.*, 9(5), 147–50 (Sept.–Oct. 1955).

6. Studies by D. H. Clarke published in *Exercise and Sport Sciences Reviews*, 1, 73–102 (1973) and by P. V. Komi, J. T. Viitasalo, R. Rauramaa & B. Vihko in the *European Journal of Applied Physiology*, 40, 45–55 (1978) have demonstrated that unilateral training produces a bilateral strength increase, which they believe is directly related to the influence of the central nervous system upon the musculature.

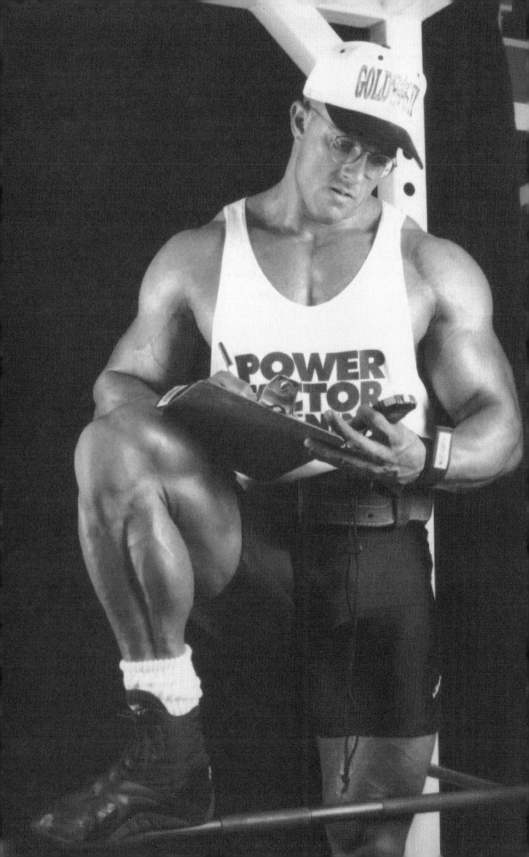

2

The Power Factor Measurement and Why You Need It

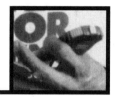

Until now your only means of gauging the value of your workouts has been by feel. If you felt particularly tired at the end of a workout, you probably assumed it was more productive than your previous one. The truth is, however, that your muscular overload might have been much less than you perceived it to be, owing to inadequate sleep the night before, consumption of the wrong foods, or some other factor. The cause of your fatigue and soreness might not have been that you subjected your muscles to a greater overload. In fact, your workout might have been a total waste of your time and effort.

As discussed in the previous chapter, there are two keys to stimulating muscle growth: (1) triggering growth by subjecting your muscles to an overload of "a great amount of work in a unit of time" and (2) making that overload progressively greater from workout to workout. Now, suppose you bench-press 150 pounds 30 times in 2 minutes today. And that's all you can do; you can't complete one more

Using Power Factor Training, you will be able to calculate ahead of time what workout you will require in order to meet your goals of increased size and strength.

rep. Then you go back to the gym next week and bench-press 150 pounds 30 times in 1½ minutes, and that's all you can do; you can't get one more rep. Both days you lifted 150 pounds for 30 repetitions. But guess what? When you do it in 1½ minutes, you are stronger.

If you don't believe me, ask Isaac Newton. It's a law of physics—the only way to lift the same amount of weight in a shorter amount of time is with a stronger "engine." If your muscles (the engine) are capable of lifting at a higher rate, they must be stronger. With conventional weight training, however, the time it takes to perform the lifting is completely ignored. In the preceding example, if you ignored time, you would enter the same results for the two workouts in your logbook. Then you'd promptly get discouraged that you were not making any progress.

THINKING IN POUNDS PER MINUTE

The Power Factor is a measurement of the total amount of weight you lift divided by the time it takes to lift it. It's measured in pounds per minute. Ask the average person in a gym what he or she bench-presses, and the reply might be, "I can bench 275." Ask a person who uses Power Factor Training the same question, and the answer might be, "I can bench 5,300 pounds per minute." Because of the laws of physics and the law of muscle fiber recruitment, the latter is a much more comprehensive measurement. Once you begin to think in pounds per minute, your training objectives and progress become crystal clear.

Using Power Factor Training, you will be able to calculate a precise Power Factor and Power Index for each exercise you perform and for your entire workout. You will also be able to calculate ahead of time what workout you

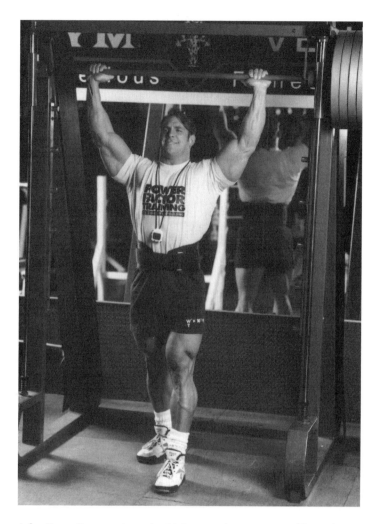

Ask a Power Factor trainer what his best standing press is, and he might say, "It's 2,800 pounds per minute."

will be required to perform next time in order to meet your goals of increased size and strength. This means that every workout can pay off in gains. If it doesn't, you'll know exactly where and why you fell short.

    You may, for example, find that your dead-lift power went down 15 percent even when your leg press power went up 21 percent. This level of precision and isolation represents a revolution in strength training.

WHAT ABOUT DISTANCE?

At this point you might be wondering why we haven't included the distance that the weight travels as part of the power calculation. There are two reasons that it is left out. Firstly, as a practical matter it is difficult to precisely measure the travel of the bar when lifting, especially in movements that involve an arc of motion, which require computations using pi (3.14159). Secondly, the length of your arms and legs isn't going to change over time, so all those distance measurements would just factor out of any comparisons that are made, leaving only differences in the weight lifted and the time. This is why we did not use horsepower or watts to measure the power that your muscles generate. A Power Factor is ideal because of its simplicity and ease of use.

DETERMINING YOUR POWER FACTOR

The purpose of calculating a Power Factor for each exercise that you perform is to provide a precise numerical measurement of your muscular output. Once you have a numerical representation of your output, you can compare the overload and effectiveness of every workout that you perform. For example, examine the two workouts described in the tables. (The time given for each total workout includes the time taken between exercises to rest and to set up the equipment. That's why the individual times do not add up to the total time.)

These two workouts are very similar, and it looks as if Workout 2 is the better one because it involves

WORKOUT 1			
Exercise	Sets	Reps	Weights
Shoulder press	2	20	150
	2	20	180
	3	15	225
	Time to Complete: 10 min.		
Lat pulldown	2	20	80
	2	20	90
	2	15	100
	Time to Complete: 11 min.		
Barbell dead lift	2	30	135
	2	20	155
	2	15	175
	Time to Complete: 14 min.		
Total Time to Complete: *41 min.			

*Includes 6 minutes to rest and to set up equipment.

WORKOUT 2			
Exercise	Sets	Reps	Weights
Shoulder press	2	20	150
	2	12	190
	2	10	245
	1	3	260
	Time to Complete: 13 min.		
Lat pulldown	2	20	90
	2	15	100
	2	10	120
	Time to Complete: 13 min.		
Barbell dead lift	2	20	155
	2	20	175
	2	15	190
	Time to Complete: 14 min.		
Total Time to Complete: *46 min.			

*Includes 6 minutes to rest and to set up equipment.

using heavier weight in every exercise. So it would stimulate more growth, right? Wrong. Actually, Workout 1 has a Power Factor that is 38 percent higher than Workout 2 and involves lifting an additional 10,135 pounds. Workout 1 represents more work in a unit of time—the key to stimulating muscle growth.

It is virtually impossible to precisely gauge that difference by feel alone. With Power Factor Training, measuring by feel is obsolete.

ANALYZING WITH THE POWER FACTOR

Let's use the Power Factor measurement to examine shoulder press performance in Workouts 1 and 2.

In Workout 1 you begin by lifting 150 pounds 20 times and perform 2 sets for a total weight lifted of

6,000 pounds. Then you perform 2 sets of 20 repetitions with 180 pounds, which adds 7,200 pounds to the total. Finally, you increase the weight on the bar to 225 pounds and perform 3 sets of 15 reps to add an additional 10,125 pounds. This brings the total amount of weight you lift to 23,325 pounds. Since it takes you 10 minutes to lift all that weight, your rate of muscular output, or Power Factor, is 2,333 pounds per minute (23,325 pounds divided by 10 minutes).

In Workout 2 you start out by lifting the same 150 pounds 20 times for 2 sets for a total weight of 6,000 pounds. Then, believing that simply adding weight alone will increase your muscular output, you increase the weight to 190 pounds and perform 2 sets of 12 reps for an additional 4,560 pounds. Pushing your limit further, you increase the weight to 245 pounds and perform 2 sets of 10 reps for an additional 4,900 pounds. Finally, still feeling strong, you increase the weight to 260 pounds and squeeze out 3 reps, bringing your total shoulder press weight to 16,240 pounds—exactly 7,085 pounds *less* than the same exercise in Workout 1! Further, since it takes 13 minutes to complete the shoulder press workout, your Power Factor drops to a comparatively dismal 1,249. That's 1,084 pounds per minute less than Workout 1—a much lower intensity of lifting.

And remember, after the last rep on each of these shoulder press workouts, you would be completely tired out. You would not be able to complete another rep. You would be "pumped," and by every sensory measure you would feel that you had given your best effort to stimulate growth. But the fact is that by using the correct combinations of weight and repetitions, Workout 1 is 38 percent more effective at generating muscular overload and the growth stimulation that goes along with it.

The same calculations reveal similar results for both of the other exercises as well as for the overall workout.

POWER FACTORS FOR WORKOUTS 1 AND 2			
Exercise	Total Weight (lb.)	Time (min.)	Power Factor
■ WORKOUT 1			
Shoulder press	23,325	10	2,333
Lat pulldown	11,400	11	1,036
Barbell dead lift	19,550	14	1,396
Total	54,275	41*	1,324
■ WORKOUT 2			
Shoulder press	16,240	13	1,249
Lat pulldown	9,000	13	692
Barbell dead lift	18,900	14	1,350
Total	44,140	46*	960

*Includes rest and set-up time.

FINDING YOUR "SWEET SPOT"

By all measures, Workout 1 is superior. The reason is that there is a relationship between the amount of weight that you put on the bar and the number of times you can lift it. It's obvious that if the weight is very light, you can do many reps but it takes a long time. If the weight is very heavy, you can only do a few reps and the lifting will be ended very fast.

For example, using the bench press, suppose that you want to determine your muscular output at the two extreme ends of this spectrum. First you select a very light weight, let's say 10 pounds, and you perform sets of 40 reps at a time. After 25 sets you are completely fatigued and cannot perform another rep. All this takes 45 minutes. You lifted 10 pounds a total of 1,000 times for a total weight of 10,000 pounds. Since it took 45 minutes to lift all that weight, your Power Factor is 222 pounds per minute. That is a low Power Factor; my grandmother could lift more than 222 pounds per minute.

Next, you test the other end of the spectrum by lifting the heaviest weight you possibly can. You put 300 pounds on the bar and, mustering all the strength you can, you perform 1 rep. You rest for a few seconds, then try to get another rep, but you just can't. Three hundred pounds is your one-rep maximum. This calculation is easy; 300 pounds in 1 minute is a Power Factor of 300 pounds per minute. It's also a very low Power Factor—a fraction of what you are capable of generating.

This example demonstrates a critically important element of strength training. If you lift too light a weight, you cannot generate a high Power Factor, yet if you lift too heavy a weight, you also cannot generate a high Power Factor. Somewhere in the middle lies your personal "sweet spot" where the perfect combination of weight, reps, and time yield your highest possible Power Factor. Finding that spot is the key to maximally efficient and productive workouts.

By the way, it varies considerably between individuals. Imagine that Subjects A and B experiment to determine how the weight they are lifting affects the number of reps they can complete in a 2-minute period. Their results are listed in the table and illustrated with the bar graphs.

As you can see in the graph for Subject A, he generates his highest Power Factor when he has 140 pounds on the bar. At that weight he can get the best ratio of total weight lifted per unit of time. That is his sweet spot.

To understand this concept is the most critical element of Power Factor Training. Subject A can put more weight on the bar—in fact, he can lift 300 pounds—but if he does, the total weight he can lift per minute is greatly decreased. Since human muscles will grow stronger and larger only when they are taxed beyond their normal operating capacity, it is crucial to discover what your operating capacity is in the first place. Subject A can

	SUBJECT A			SUBJECT B		
Weight on Bar (lb.)	Total Reps	Total Weight (lb)	Power Factor (lb./min.)	Total Reps	Total Weight (lb.)	Power Factor (lb./min.)
40	120	4,800	2,400	120	4,800	2,400
60	108	6,480	3,240	111	6,660	3,330
80	96	7,680	3,840	102	8,160	4,080
100	84	8,400	4,200	93	9,300	4,650
120	72	8,640	4,320	84	10,080	5,040
140	63	8,820	4,410	80	11,200	5,600
160	54	8,640	4,320	76	12,160	6,080
180	45	8,100	4,050	72	12,960	6,480
200	36	7,200	3,600	68	13,600	6,800
220	29	6,380	3,190	64	14,080	7,040
240	22	5,280	2,640	50	12,000	6,000
260	15	3,900	1,950	36	9,360	4,680
280	8	2,240	1,120	16	4,480	2,240
300	2	600	300	4	1,200	600

lift 280 pounds 8 times in 2 minutes, and it will take everything he has to perform those reps, but it is nowhere near his muscle's full capacity for lifting. Therefore, while that routine might generate some adaptive response, it is very inefficient compared to him lifting 140 pounds 63 times in the same 2-minute period.

This is a well-settled principle of physics. An engine that lifts 4,410 pounds per minute has to be more powerful than an engine that lifts 1,120 pounds per minute.

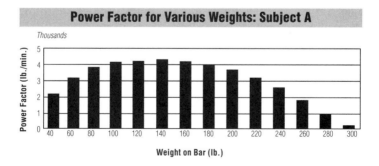

Power Factor for Various Weights: Subject A

Your muscle fibers are the engine; nothing else does the lifting.

Subject B demonstrates the variation that occurs among individuals. His highest Power Factor is achieved when he has 220 pounds on the bar. He can put more or less weight on the bar, but his personal sweet spot is at 220 pounds.

Why? Many factors contribute to the ability of muscle fibers to activate and to the power they generate. Some of them we know, and some of them we are yet to fully understand. Where the muscle physically attaches to the bone relative to the joint has a profound effect on leverage. The neural pathways between the brain and muscles have varying efficiencies in individuals. The body's ability to supply and process ATP to the muscles varies between individuals, as do the mix of slow-twitch and fast-twitch fibers in each muscle. The complex cocktail of blood, oxygen, amino acids, and hormones that supply the entire process has nearly infinite possibilities of variation. But here is the good news. All you have to concentrate on is developing your highest possible Power Factor for each exercise, because it gives a clear indication of what is delivering the most overload to your muscles and what is not.

You can't take blood samples and tissue biopsies after each exercise that you perform in order to analyze which technique is generating the greatest metabolic changes.

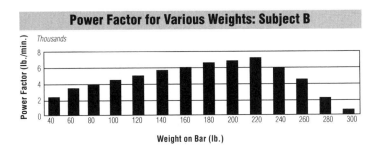

You can't place your body in an MRI machine during each exercise to see what area of a muscle is activated by a particular exercise. You can't perform a CAT scan on your brain to determine what neural pathways are being activated by today's workout. But you don't need to! If your Power Factor is 6,500 pounds per minute this workout, and last workout it was 5,600 pounds per minute, then you are absolutely, positively generating more output from your muscles. And who cares if it's because of hormone secretion or neural pathways or both? All these systems work together anyway, so isolating one or the other through complex testing does not really provide any practical benefit to the athlete who just wants results. Train by the numbers, and everything else will take care of itself.

SIMPLE ARITHMETIC

As you perform your workout, all you need to do is keep track of how many minutes it takes to do each exercise (bench press, dead lifts, shrugs, etc.), how much weight you're using, and how many reps and sets you do with each weight. Record this information on the Workout Record form.

Caution: Warm up completely before you start to time your workout. To warm up, utilize only the barest amount of energy and movement required to thoroughly warm up the joints, muscles, and connective tissues of the body parts you're going to be training, and perform only enough sets to obtain a slight pump and to achieve viscosity in the joints. For example, start out with just the empty bar you're about to utilize and perform 1–2 sets of fairly high (20–30) repetitions with it. Then add what for you is some appreciable resistance and perform 2 more sets of moderate reps (about 10–20). Add weight again and, if needed, perform 1–2 more sets. You should be adequately warmed up by this point and ready to start your real sets. For the sake of consistency, try to use the same warm-up routine every time.

Here's how to use the Workout Record:

❶ Enter the time of day that you begin your workout. This will be used to calculate your overall performance. In all cases you should be sure to fully warm up before starting the clock on your workout. You should first perform your warm-up, taking as long as you like, then start timing your Power Factor Training. Your warm-up should never be counted as part of your Power Factor. Doing so will lead to an incentive to use heavy weights too quickly, ultimately causing injury. Warm up completely before you start to time your workout.

❷ Enter the time of day that you finish your workout.

❸ Subtract your Start Time from your Finish Time to get the Total Time of your workout. Always express this in minutes only (for instance, 95 minutes, not 1 hour and 35 minutes). Enter this time at the top of the page and as the Total Time on the last line. The Total Time includes *all* the time used from the beginning of your workout (but not the warm-up) to the end. It includes rests between sets and rests between exercises and the time you spent changing weights and getting a drink of water. It is *not* just the sum of your individual exercise times.

❹ Calculate the total weight lifted per set by simple arithmetic. For example, if you perform 20 repetitions with 105 pounds, you multiply the two numbers to get 2,100 pounds. If you do 2 sets at that weight, you multiply by 2 to get 4,200 pounds. Put another way, you've lifted 105 pounds 40 times for a total weight lifted of 4,200 pounds. Again, do not include weight lifted during your warm-up. The warm-up itself should not degenerate into a workout.

❺ Calculate the total weight per exercise by adding the row of subtotals.

❻ Measure the exercise time from the time you start each individual exercise to the time you finish. It should always include the time you rest between sets. It should not include warm-up time. You will find a stopwatch very helpful for measuring this time.

❼ Calculate the Power Factor by dividing the total weight by the time it took to lift it. So, if you lift 16,730 pounds in 7.5 minutes, your Power Factor is 2,231 pounds per minute ($16,730 \div 7.5 = 2,231$). This is the power output of your muscles. On average, every minute you lifted 2,231 pounds. If you can increase that number on your next workout, you will know that you have increased the overload and gained strength.

❽ To calculate the Power Index, multiply the total weight by the Power Factor, then divide the product by 1,000,000.

❾ Calculate the total weight for the workout by adding the total weight from each exercise (in this example, $16,730 + 13,040 + 8,940 + 72,785 + 72,680 = 184,175$ pounds). This number represents the total amount of weight you lifted during your workout.

26   *Power Factor Training*

WORKOUT RECORD   Date: __7__ / __16__ / __97__

❶ Start Time: __8:05 A.M.__   **❷** Finish Time: __8:51 A.M.__   **❸** Total Time: __46 MIN.__

■ Exercise: DEAD LIFT

Weight Reps Sets	Weight Reps Sets	Weight Reps Sets	Weight Reps Sets	Weight Reps Sets	Weight Reps Sets
105×20×2	135×20×2	155×20×1	155×26×1	× ×	× ×
Subtotal = 4,200 lb.	Subtotal = 5,400 lb.	Subtotal = 3,100 lb.	Subtotal = 4,030 lb.	Subtotal = lb.	Subtotal = lb.

❹ *Exercise 1:*   Total Weight __16,730__ lb.   Time: __7½__ min.   Power Factor __2,231__ lb./min.   Power Index __37.3__

■ Exercise: BENCH PRESS

Weight Reps Sets	Weight Reps Sets	Weight Reps Sets	Weight Reps Sets	Weight Reps Sets	Weight Reps Sets
120×15×2	140×15×2	160×13×1	160×11×1	175×8×1	× ×
Subtotal = 3,600 lb.	Subtotal = 4,200 lb.	Subtotal = 2,080 lb.	Subtotal = 1,760 lb.	Subtotal = 1,400 lb.	Subtotal = lb.

Exercise 2:   Total Weight __13,040__ lb.   Time: __8¼__ min.   Power Factor __1,581__ lb./min.   Power Index __20.6__

■ Exercise: LAT PULLDOWNS

Weight Reps Sets	Weight Reps Sets	Weight Reps Sets	Weight Reps Sets	Weight Reps Sets	Weight Reps Sets
60×18×2	70×18×2	80×19×1	90×16×1	100×13×1	× ×
Subtotal = 2,160 lb.	Subtotal = 2,520 lb.	Subtotal = 1,520 lb.	Subtotal = 1,440 lb.	Subtotal = 1,300 lb.	Subtotal = lb.

Exercise 3:   Total Weight __8,940__ lb.   Time: __6¾__ min.   Power Factor __1,324__ lb./min.   Power Index __11.8__

■ Exercise: LEG PRESS

Weight Reps Sets	Weight Reps Sets	Weight Reps Sets	Weight Reps Sets	Weight Reps Sets	Weight Reps Sets
300×20×1	400×20×2	450×20×2	500×23×1	525×21×1	540×19×1
Subtotal = 6,000 lb.	Subtotal = 16,000 lb.	Subtotal = 18,000 lb.	Subtotal = 11,500 lb.	Subtotal = 11,025 lb.	Subtotal = 10,260 lb.

Exercise 4:   Total Weight __72,785__ lb.   Time: __7½__ min.   Power Factor __9,705__ lb./min.   Power Index __706__

■ Exercise: TOE PRESS

Weight Reps Sets	Weight Reps Sets	Weight Reps Sets	Weight Reps Sets	Weight Reps Sets	Weight Reps Sets
350×20×1	400×20×2	450×20×2	500×24×1	525×20×1	540×17×1
Subtotal = 7,000 lb.	Subtotal = 16,000 lb.	Subtotal = 18,000 lb.	Subtotal = 12,000 lb.	Subtotal = 10,500 lb.	Subtotal = 9,180 lb.

Exercise 5:   Total Weight __72,680__ lb.   Time: __7__ min.   Power Factor __10,383__ lb./min.   Power Index __755__

OVERALL WORKOUT: Total Weight __184,175__ lb.   Time: __46__ min.   Power Factor __4,004__ lb./min.   Power Index __737__

Exercise Subtotal = Weight × Reps × Sets   ■ Power Factor = lb./min.   ■ Power Index = Total Weight × Power Factor ÷ 1,000,000

⑩ To find the Power Factor for the overall workout, divide the total weight by the total time. In this case, 184,175 ÷ 46 = 4,004.

⑪ To calculate the Power Index for your workout, multiply the total weight by the Power Factor, then divide the product by 1,000,000. In this example, 184,175 × 4,004 ÷ 1,000,000 = 737.

Filling in this form will give you all of the data that you need to measure the effectiveness of this workout, engineer the next workout, and keep your progress steady and consistent while avoiding overtraining.

EVERYTHING IS RELATIVE

The Power Factor measurement was adopted because of its simplicity. However, in some respects it is a relative measurement. In other words, as stated earlier, it can only be used as a comparison of similar workouts. For example, if you perform full-range exercises today, strong-range exercises tomorrow, and "super slow" exercises the next day, the associated Power Factors won't mean much when compared. However, if you were to adopt full-range training or super slow or virtually any other method for a few weeks at a time, your Power Factor numbers would still be an excellent way to compare the intensity of each workout and to ensure progressive overload. In fact, they would be indispensable.

The same proviso holds for comparing Power Factors of different individuals. If one person moves the bar farther or deliberately moves slower, then he may have a lower Power Factor number than someone else despite actually being stronger. Such comparisons are irrelevant, so don't spend any time worrying about them. Just work on improving your numbers.

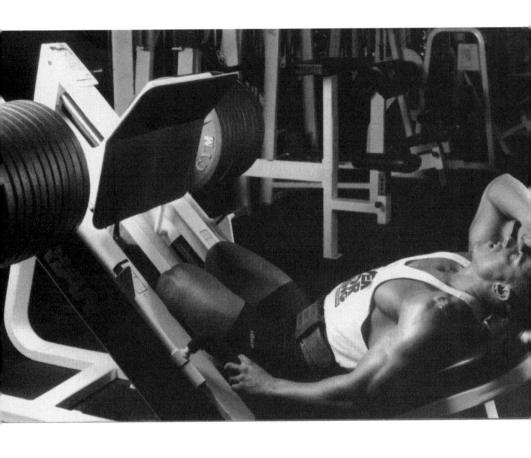

3

The Power Index

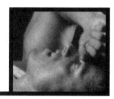

The human body is a wonder of engineering. It has a remarkable variety of automatic survival and protection mechanisms that we are only beginning to understand. Breathe in some bacteria, and one mechanism goes to work. Cut your hand, and a different mechanism kicks in. Jump into cold water or get under the hot sun, and your body immediately goes to work compensating for the stress and sending survival signals to your brain. One of those safety systems prevents you from working out too strenuously. Call it fatigue, muscular failure, or running out of gas, it's what protects you from exercising to the point of putting too much stress on your body's recuperative abilities.

Call it fatigue, muscular failure, or running out of gas, it's what protects you from exercising to the point of putting too much stress on your body's recuperative abilities.

ALPHA STRENGTH AND BETA STRENGTH: TWO WAYS TO GROW

If you think of lifting weight as performing work the way a machine does, then there are two measures of that machine's strength or power. One is the rate of lifting that it can achieve, like 20 tons per hour. The other measure is the amount of time that the machine can sustain that rate of work, like 4 hours or 24 hours before needing to be shut down. The human body has the same two forms of power, but there are protection mechanisms that try to prevent you from operating at their extreme limits. That's why you can perform a set to failure but after only a few seconds' rest perform more reps with the same weight. Some people, after only sixty to ninety seconds of rest, can exactly duplicate the first set to failure. That means they have much more strength capacity but do not tap into all of it in only one set.

This phenomenon of hitting an initial wall of fatigue that can be overcome with brief rest is just one more protection mechanism of your body. It keeps extra muscular energy in reserve just in case it's required in the near future—for example, in one or two minutes. If you never use that reserve amount of strength, it will never grow to a higher level because it doesn't have to.

We call these two forms of human power alpha strength and beta strength. Alpha strength is akin to a snapshot in that it gives a measurement of your rate of lifting for a moment in time, perhaps a minute or two. Beta strength is more like a motion picture that can measure how long you can sustain your alpha strength. There is a subtle but extremely important difference.

To illustrate the point, consider that the 1995 edition of the *Guinness Book of Records* lists John "Jack" Atherton as setting a record by bench-pressing 1,134,828 total pounds in 12 hours. That's a rate of lifting of 1,576 pounds per minute, a rate nearly anyone reading this could duplicate, but he sustained that rate for 12 hours! I can already hear some of you saying, "Twelve hours? That's aerobic exercise!" However, while there is no question that sustaining activity for that long is aerobic in nature, the fact is that it was his muscles that lifted that million plus pounds, not his well-developed heart and lungs.

On the other hand, the Bill Kazmaiers and Anthony Clarks of the world can generate the highest alpha strength. A 700-pound-plus bench press or a 900-pound-plus squat represents an astronomically high rate of instantaneous muscular output that the human body will sustain for only a very short period of time.

Here is the most important fact for bodybuilders in all of this analysis: both forms of strength build muscle mass. Mass is the ingredient that every bodybuilder is after, but how many realize that if they are not making progress with one method of strength building, they can try another? Most bodybuilders don't really care about strength per se, they just want to increase it as a means to gaining more mass. But understanding how strength manifests in the human body can help you measure and guarantee your progress.

If strength can be increased in two ways, then we need to measure it in two ways. We measure alpha strength with the formula $\frac{W}{t}$, or total weight (W) divided by total time (t). The formula for beta strength is $\frac{W^2}{t} \times 10^{-6}$, or total weight (W) squared divided by total time (t) divided by 1,000,000. These two measurements are the Power Factor and Power Index, respectively. The Power Factor measures the intensity of your lifting (for example, a bench press rate of 2,500 pounds per minute). In contrast, the Power Index is a relative measurement of how long you can sustain a given rate of lifting. If you sustain 2,500 pounds per minute for 3.5 minutes, your Power Index is 21.9. If you sustain it for 11 minutes, your Power Index is 68.8.[1] Please notice that in both cases your Power Factor is the same 2,500 pounds per minute; there is no difference in alpha strength.

In a strict sense, any discussion of how strong or powerful a person is depends on the period of time over which

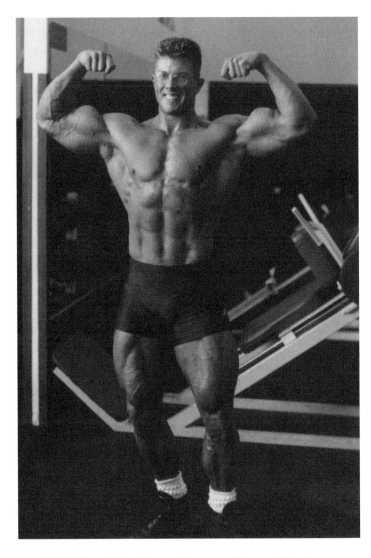

Most bodybuilders don't really care about strength per se. They just want to increase it as a means to gaining more mass.

we are measuring. Over a 10-second period, Anthony Clark is king. Over 12 hours it's the aforementioned Jack Atherton. I wonder which of the two would be stronger over a 2-hour period?

We frequently talk to frustrated bodybuilders who are making no progress because they have fallen into the trap of performing only 1 set, 3 sets, 30 reps, or whatever. What they don't realize is that they are always measuring their progress on a fixed, usually short, time scale. In effect, they measure progress by alpha strength only and never really tax that reserve sustained strength, their beta strength. All of them could make new progress by measuring their beta strength and making sure that it progressively increases from workout to workout.

WHY YOU NEED THE POWER INDEX

There are two ways that you can get stronger. If you lift 2,000 pounds per minute today and last workout you lifted only 1,700 pounds per minute, then you are stronger. However, if you lifted 1,700 pounds per minute for 5 minutes last workout and this workout you lifted 1,700 pounds per minute for 7 minutes, you are also stronger, even though your Power Factor did not change. Why? Physics, again. If an engine (your muscles) can continue lifting at a certain rate but for a longer period of time, it has to be stronger. You can't get something for nothing; more work done requires more strength.

As your Power Factor Training progresses, you will become familiar with the two ways to achieve higher Power Factors. Basically, you can either lift more total weight, or you can lift the same weight in a shorter period of time. While both achievements represent an increase in muscular output, the tactic of constantly trying to work out in less time has obvious limitations. For one thing, the quicker your workout pace, the greater the likelihood of producing an injury. Also, constantly reducing the time of your workout will ignore beta strength training. Remember, being able to lift at the same rate but for a longer period of time also is an indication of increased strength.

You can achieve an extremely high Power Factor rating by performing certain exercises over a very short period of time. For example, suppose that you perform 6 calf raises with 500 pounds in 6 seconds. Your Power Factor, based on the average pounds per minute, would be a staggering 30,000 pounds per minute! Of course, you really didn't lift 30,000 pounds, nor did you work out for 1 minute, but your rate of lifting for $\frac{1}{10}$ minute would be 30,000 pounds per minute! This is the limitation of looking at Power Factor numbers in isolation. Theoretically, you could increase your Power Factor every workout by using this tactic, but you'd be cheating yourself. This is where the Power Index comes into play.

The Power Index is a mathematical function of the total weight lifted and the Power Factor. It simultaneously reflects both the total weight you lift and the rate of your lifting. Since the Power Index is calculated by multiplying the total weight (W) by the Power Factor ($\frac{W}{t}$), the weight component of your workout is actually squared. This produces a very large number, which is then divided by one million in order to make it more manageable. Using the example of six 500-pound calf raises in 6 seconds (30,000 Power Factor), the Power Index would be just 90 (that is, 3,000 lb. × 30,000 lb./min. ÷ 1,000,000). By way of contrast, during the development of this system, we were routinely achieving Power Indexes in calf raises of well over 4,500!

Because calculating the Power Index involves squaring the total weight lifted, the Power Index is graphed on a logarithmic scale. Consequently, a modest increase in strength can yield a large increase in the Power Index. These increases can be disproportionate both in raw numbers and in percentages (in fact, you shouldn't use percentages). The only important element is that the trend be

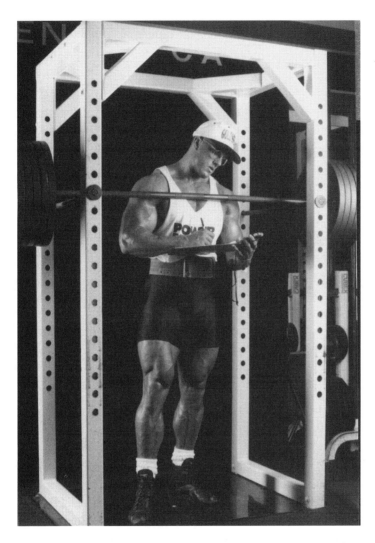

As your Power Factor Training progresses, you will become familiar with the two ways to achieve higher numbers.

in an upward direction. That is an indication of improvement and enough to guide you in the direction of progress.

You can't cheat the Power Index. The only way to make big gains in your Power Index is to work toward lifting at a high Power Factor and to keep it up for as long as you can. In short, you must maintain a high muscular output (pounds per minute) for as long as possible. The Power Index gives you a clear indication of whether or not your strength is increasing by measuring your capacity to continue lifting at the same rate but for a longer time. The Power Factor gives you a clear indication of whether or not your strength is increasing by measuring your capacity to lift at a higher rate.

Those are the only two ways your muscles (or any engine) can get stronger. By monitoring these two numbers, you will have instant feedback as to what exercises and techniques yield results and which do not. You can also instantly spot overtraining or a plateau. The efficiency of this system is what makes it revolutionary. As you will see, the gains you stand to make from using it will be spectacular.

SISCO'S LAWS OF BODYBUILDING

Momentary Intensity $(I_m = \frac{W}{t})$
1. In the realm of human exertion, there are actually two forms of strength, which we refer to as alpha strength and beta strength. The measure of alpha strength is what we call the Power Factor (*PF*). Momentary intensity is expressed mathematically as $I_m = \frac{W}{t}$, where W is the total weight lifted in pounds and t is the total time in minutes. A high intensity of muscular overload is one of the indispensable conditions of triggering muscle growth. It therefore behooves us, in the interest of greater precision and a more exact science, to have a means of quantifying that intensity.

    When we measure momentary intensity with the Power Factor (*PF*) measurement, we can identify and increase alpha strength. For example, if a trainee performs 20 reps with 200 pounds in 2 minutes, he has lifted a total weight of 4,000 pounds for a Power Factor of 2,000 pounds per minute (20 × 200 lb. ÷ 2 min. = 2,000 lb./min.). If that same trainee, next time in the gym, performs 20 reps with 200 pounds in only 1.5 minutes, his Power Factor increases to 2,667 pounds per minute (20 × 200 lb. ÷ 1.5 min. = 2,667 lb./min.). This increase in Power Factor accurately reflects the trainee's ability to perform the exercise at a higher intensity. Without this measurement, on both workout days the trainee would simply enter "20 reps at 200 pounds" or "2 sets of 10 reps at 200 pounds" in his logbook and promptly get discouraged that he made "no progress" when, in fact, he made great progress.

2. *The momentary intensity* (I_m) *of any exercise is inversely proportionate to the duration* (D) *over which it can be sustained. In plain English, the longer the duration of an exercise or workout, the lower the momentary intensity must be.* This law is self-evident. You can perform more reps before reaching fatigue with 10 pounds than with 100 pounds, but it takes longer.

Volumetric Intensity $(I_v = \frac{W^2}{t} \times 10^{-6})$

3. We measure beta strength in terms of the Power Index through volumetric intensity (I_v). Mathematically, it is expressed as $I_v = \frac{W^2}{t} \times 10^{-6}$, where W is the total weight lifted in pounds and t is the total time in minutes.

   When we measure intensity with the Power Index, we can identify an increase in beta strength. For example, suppose a trainee performs an exercise with a Power Factor of 1,500 pounds per minute (his momentary intensity) and is able to sustain that rate of lifting for 3 minutes before he is at failure. Next time in the gym, he still has a Power Factor of 1,500 pounds per minute but is able to sustain it for 4.5 minutes before he reaches failure. If we look only at his Power Factor (momentary intensity), he has made no progress. However, it is obvious that he is stronger, since he can sustain the same high level of muscular output for a longer period of time. This ability is his beta strength, and it is measured with the Power Index. His initial Power Index is 6.8, and his second Power Index is 10.1. This increase in Power Index accurately reflects the trainee's ability to sustain the intensity for a long period of time.

Frequency of Training Is Inversely Proportional to Volumetric Intensity

4. The body needs time to recover, so your Power Index will be lower when you train more frequently (other things being equal). In scientific terms, the volumetric intensity of a workout is inversely proportional to the frequency of training, due to the trainee's finite recovery capacity. Stated mathematically, $F = \frac{R}{I_v}$, where F is the frequency of training, R is the trainee's recovery capacity, and I_v is the volumetric intensity of the workout.

   Human physiology is such that while a person can increase his or her muscular strength by a factor of at least 300 percent, his or her supporting organs will not increase their functional capacity at the same time or to the same degree. For example, there is a limit on how much cellular waste your kidneys can process in, say, a twenty-four-hour period. If you double your strength through weight lifting, your kidneys will not also double their efficiency or size so they can process more in twenty-four hours. Since organs like the kidneys, liver, pancreas, and others have relatively fixed rates of performing their functions and will not grow larger and more efficient with more use, it is necessary to give them more time to complete their jobs as you get stronger. The fact is, humans have the ability to perform muscular work at a higher rate than their supporting organs can replenish themselves.

At this time we have no unit of measurement for recovery capacity (R), and it certainly must vary enormously among individuals, as well as in the same person from time to time. For example, when ill or when getting over an illness, you would have a greatly diminished recovery capacity. What is important to remember is the principle that, because of a relatively fixed and finite recovery capacity, your frequency of training (F) must decrease as your volumetric intensity (I_v) increases.

This law prevents consistent progress when using a fixed training schedule. In other words, if you always train three days per week, you will reach a point where your volumetric intensity (or Power Index) cannot be progressively increased. Without progressive overload, there can be no new growth stimulation. You must decrease training frequency if you want to increase intensity. Like gravity, it's the law.

THE MILLION-POUND WORKOUT

If you would like an idea of how dramatic a subject's results can be when Sisco's laws are properly obeyed and applied, consider this example. When we first began the development of Power Factor Training in 1992, our performances were nothing spectacular, to be sure. A typical workout of shoulders and arms, consisting of three different exercises, yielded an overall workout performance of a 343 Power Factor and a 5.3 Power Index. Similarly, a chest, back, and legs workout, consisting of three different exercises, yielded an 848 Power Factor and a 36 Power Index.

At this point the twofold benefit of (1) exercising in the strongest range of motion combined with (2) exact monitoring of muscular power output (to avoid both wasted effort and overtraining) led to an explosion of improvement. We were able to add more exercises to our workouts and more weight to each exercise. After fifty-two days on the program (consisting of only sixteen workouts), our shoulder and arm workouts yielded a Power Factor of 3,948 with a Power Index of 1,387. Our chest, back, and leg workouts now yielded a Power Factor of 6,423 and a Power Index of 3,713. Workouts that had begun with bench presses, shrugs, and leg presses of 175 pounds, 135 pounds, and 450 pounds, respectively, were now up to an astounding 500 pounds, 540 pounds, and 1,325 pounds, respectively! And these were not single-repetition weights. These were "sweet spot" workout weights that we used to perform many sets of multiple repetitions.

On the fortieth day of the program, we arranged a special test of the system. We took a couple of days of extra rest and were careful to carb up with the proper foods. We designed a special workout that combined upper and lower body parts and performed, in effect, a whole-body workout. We used the bench press, dead lift, barbell shrug, leg press, and toe press and, in 131 minutes, we each lifted 1,000,375 pounds. This yielded a Power Factor of 7,636 pounds per minute and a Power Index of 7,639. By way of comparison, that Power Factor is equivalent to lifting two Lincoln Continentals every minute! Further, we kept up that pace for 2 hours and 11 minutes. This clearly and convincingly demonstrates the fantastic muscle- and strength-building capacity and efficiency of this training system.

NOTE

1. Mathematically speaking, the reason a longer time generates a bigger Power Index is that as the time increases, you lift a larger total weight to get an equal Power Factor:

2,500 lb./1 min. = 8,750 lb./3.5 min. = 27,500 lb./11 min.

Since computing the Power Index requires that you square the weight, the difference in total weight makes a tremendous difference in the Power Index:

$$Pi_1 = PF \times W_1 \div 1,000,000 = 2,500 \times 8,750 \div 1,000,000 = 21.9$$
$$Pi_2 = PF \times W_2 \div 1,000,000 = 2,500 \times 27,500 \div 1,000,000 = 68.8$$

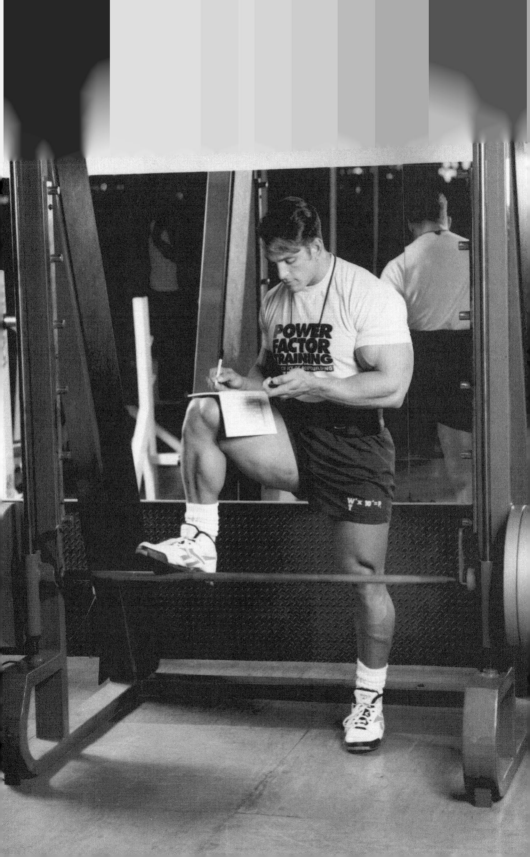

Monitoring for Optimum Results

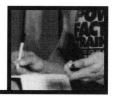

4

Never perform a blind workout wherein you just lift weights without regard to the reps, sets, and exact time taken for each exercise. It's a wasted workout. Even if the intensity is sufficient to stimulate some new muscle growth, you'll have no way of knowing what intensity you need next time you're in the gym. It's sloppy, and there is no excuse for it.

Being aware of the time it takes to perform an exercise is critical to making efficient progress.

The most significant ramification of the innovation of the Power Factor and Power Index is the ability, for the first time in the history of strength training, to provide a simple and mathematically precise indication of muscular output. Once this ability is established, it permits the most effective and efficient way to objectively measure your progress. Theories, myths, folklore, and science can all be put to the ultimate laboratory tests: How much overload does it deliver to the muscles? Does it develop greater strength? How much? How fast?

And this is just the tip of the iceberg. Henceforth, every factor that contributes to or detracts from your progress also can be measured.

You will be able to accurately measure the effect of more or fewer reps, more or fewer sets, heavier or lighter weight, longer or shorter workouts, extra days off between workouts, use of different supplements, other variations in your diet, and more. In the domain of body-building, powerlifting, or any other form of strength training, such instant and precise assessment is nothing short of revolutionary. No longer is it necessary for the strength athlete to measure progress by "feel" or "instinct." And all the equipment you need to unleash this powerful new technology is a logbook and a stop-watch—common items in virtually every other sport and yet so crucial in determining and plotting progress.

Could you imagine, for example, an Olympic miler trying to monitor his or her progress by "feel" or "instinct" while experimenting with running techniques like wind sprints, intervals, running hills, and so on, never measuring progress by using a stopwatch? Never having any tangible, objective measure of the effects of his or her training techniques nor of improvement from one month to the next? Yet this is exactly the type of low-tech methodology that strength athletes have always used.

WRITE IT DOWN

During your Power Factor Training workouts, you will record on the Workout Record form the time, sets, reps, and weights that you lifted. After you perform a workout, record your results for each individual exercise and your overall workout performance on the Exercise/Workout Performance Record form.

The only calculation you need to carry out on the Exercise/Workout Performance Record forms is the per-centage of change from workout to workout. To find the percentage of change, use this simple method:

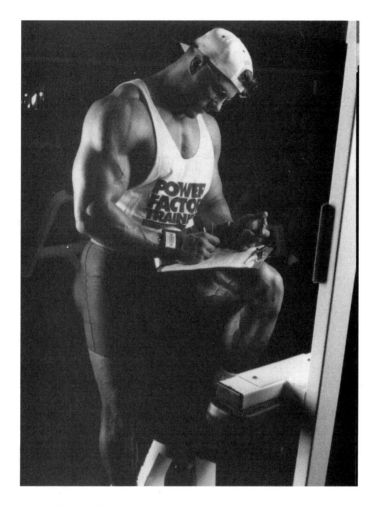

*Use the Workout Record form to record the time, sets, reps, and weights
you lifted.*

1. New Number − Old Number = Difference
2. Difference ÷ Old Number × 100% = % Change

For example, suppose your Power Factor goes from
1,675 to 1,890. Find the percentage of change:

$$1,890 - 1,675 = 215$$
$$215 \div 1,675 \times 100\% = 12.8\%$$

EXERCISE/WORKOUT PERFORMANCE RECORD

■ **Exercise:**

Date	Total Weight	% Change	Power Factor	% Change	Power Index	+ or – Change

PLAN AHEAD

One of the most powerful aspects of Power Factor Training is its capability to permit you to plan a workout ahead of time in order to achieve a target goal. The calculations necessary to do this are still fairly simple, and

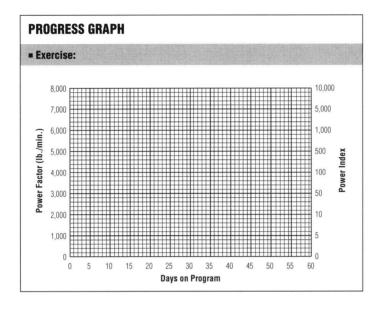

we encourage you to familiarize yourself with the technique, as it is the key to guaranteeing that every workout is effective, efficient, and progressive. As you do so, keep in mind that the two keys to maximum overload are total weight and time. Those are the only two factors that you will adjust in your workouts.

For example, using the bench press numbers from the Workout Record entry on page 26, we see that the total weight lifted was 13,040 pounds, and the Power Factor was 1,581 pounds per minute. You can find the time it took you to perform this exercise by looking at the Workout Record or by dividing the total weight by the Power Factor ($13,040 \div 1,581 = 8.25$). Now, suppose you set a goal of achieving a 20 percent increase in your total weight and a 10 percent increase in your Power Factor the next time you perform the bench press. Simply follow these steps:

1. Add 20 percent to 13,040 pounds ($13,040 \times 1.20 = 15,648$).

2. Add 10 percent to 1,581 pounds per minute (1,581 × 1.10 = 1,739).
3. Divide the goal total weight by the goal Power Factor. Your result is the time (in minutes) allowed to perform the lifting (15,648 ÷ 1,739 = 9.00).

As a result of having made these simple calculations, you now know exactly what you have to do in your next workout to ensure that your muscular output (overload) is higher: you have to lift 15,650 pounds in 9 minutes (see table). You can achieve your goal total weight simply by increasing your bench press Power Factor (pounds per minute) by adding an extra set or more reps to each set or by using a heavier weight so that the total will be 15,650 pounds. As you work out, keep an eye on your stopwatch to ensure that you don't go over the 9 minutes you've set as your target time, and you will be certain that your Power Factor and Power Index have increased.

Here is one of the most important things to keep in mind. Ideally, no two workouts should ever be the same, because each time you return to the gym, you are a different man (or woman). If your last workout was properly engineered, it stimulated muscle growth, and if you allowed yourself the required time for recovery and growth, you are a stronger person when you return to the gym. Therefore, performing the same workout as last time is useless. Since your muscles are now capable of more output, the old workout will not trigger any growth

COMPONENTS OF A POWER FACTOR TRAINING GOAL			
	Total Weight (lb.)	Power Factor (lb./min.)	Time (min.)
Current Performance	13,040	1,581	8.25
Goal	15,650	1,739	9.00

response. Get it? That's what progressive overload is all about. Do the same workout every time, and you get nowhere; engineer an ever-increasing overload, and you get steadily stronger. The "engineering" is done with the Power Factor and Power Index numbers.

Goals can be set for one or all exercises you perform and for your total workout as well. It is difficult to overstate the tremendous value of this ability to plan every workout to ensure that it is productive. This is the element of Power Factor Training that creates its efficiency and is the reason that such a high percentage of its trainees can work out once a week or less and still see consistent improvement all the way to the optimum-level muscularity that they desire. Every workout is a positive step toward the trainee's ultimate goal. Compare this to the old systems of everyone following a prescribed chart of exercises for six weeks, then switching to another chart for six more weeks, and so on, with every trainee using the same daily schedule and repetition schemes regardless of the huge amount of variation among individuals (remember the sweet spot?). Power Factor Training gives you the ability to engineer every workout that you perform to be maximally productive for your particular physiology.

GRAPH YOUR RESULTS

This technique of scientifically planning your goals ahead of time and monitoring your results permits the highest possible muscular overload each workout and the greatest possible gains in size and strength. You will be readily able to see your progress by plotting your Power Factor and Power Index numbers on the graph paper located in your logbook. The graph shown here reflects one subject's change in his overall workout Power Index during a period of eighteen workouts over sixty days. The trend

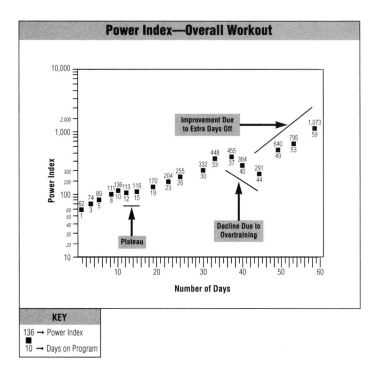

Power Index—Overall Workout

KEY

136 → Power Index
■
10 → Days on Program

that you should see on your graph is a consistent increase in your Power Factor and Power Index numbers, both on individual exercises and on your workout.

As in the example, a workout may not always yield an increase, and you may even see a decrease in your numbers. This, as you will discover, can be caused by a variety of circumstances. You may have worked out after eating too few carbohydrates or after having had too little sleep or when unable to concentrate due to stress. However, the number-one cause of a prolonged inability to improve is overtraining. Much more will be said about this crucial point later in this book, but for now it is critical to remember that muscular growth takes place only after you have recovered from your last workout. The recovery and growth processes require time to complete themselves. If you do not allow for this fact, your muscles cannot grow.

The sample graph shows steady progress on a Monday, Wednesday, Friday schedule, but by the twelfth day a decline in the Power Index occurred. By switching to a schedule of two days per week, the trainee gave his metabolism the required time, not only to recover, but to increase muscle mass. On a twice-a-week schedule, tremendous gains were made up to the thirty-third day. At this point, rather than just hitting a plateau, muscular output decreased sharply. Once again, this was corrected by adding more time off between workouts. As expected, the Power Index again showed a tremendous improvement.

You will note that the change in Power Index from Day 1 to Day 59 is enormous. This reflects a great increase in both the total amount of weight lifted and the rate of lifting (pounds/minutes). Such numerical gains can be achieved only through a great increase in muscular strength and therefore create a corresponding increase in muscular size.

Importantly, even subtle changes in the athlete's performance can be quickly and graphically identified and corrected through proper alterations in the workout and/or the training schedule. Power Factor Training identifies and prevents the chronic plateaus and overtraining that plague strength athletes who rely on the old, crude gauges of feel and instinct to measure their performance.

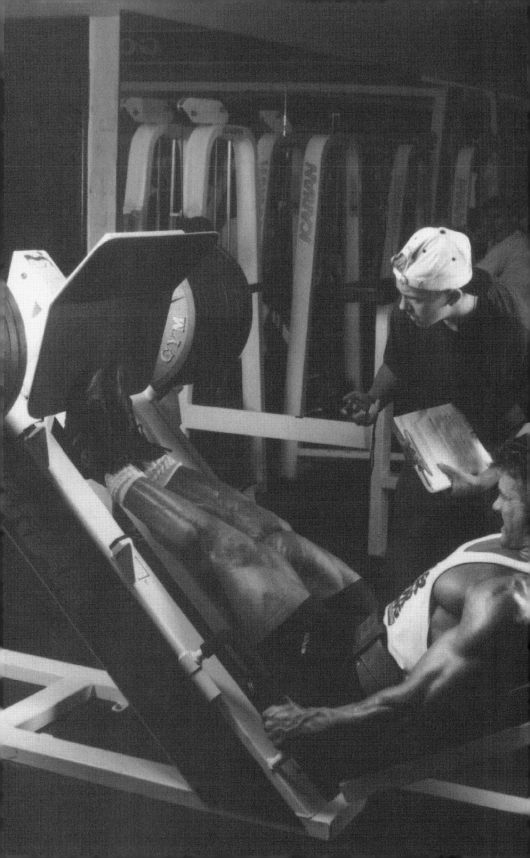

5

Maximum Overload for Maximum Gains

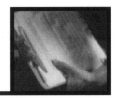

The amount of overload you can impose on a muscle is directly correlated with how much size and strength it can acquire. The greater the overload imposed, the greater the potential size and strength increase. Specific demands imposed upon the body result in specific physiological adjustments. This fact forms a concept central to exercise physiology known as the principle of specific adaptation to imposed demands (SAID). According to the SAID principles, if training is to be performed for the purpose of stimulating increases in strength and size, then the demands must be of a specific nature— namely, peak overload and maximum muscular output.

However, as our bodies adapt to a certain level of resistance by developing larger and stronger muscles, the overload in our workouts must be increased if further growth is to be achieved. This cause-and-effect relationship has been labeled the progressive overload principle, which states that in order to grow progressively larger muscles, the skeletal

The greater the overload imposed, the greater the potential increases in muscle size and strength.

muscles must be routinely subjected to ever-increasing demands. This is not only one of the most basic principles of strength development, it's also the cornerstone of Power Factor Training.

THE LAW OF MUSCLE FIBER RECRUITMENT

As far as building muscular mass is concerned, the sole objective is muscle fiber recruitment. The more muscle fibers recruited, the more activated; the more activated, the greater the growth stimulation. It therefore stands to reason that the more muscle fibers called into play or made to contract against resistance, the more muscle fibers will be stimulated to hypertrophy, or grow larger.

It was demonstrated clinically in 1973 that, at light loads, slow-twitch fibers contract and are capable of sustaining repeated contractions at this relatively low intensity. Since these fibers are weaker, they're not suited to a higher intensity of effort or overload. If a greater load is imposed upon the muscle, a progressive recruitment of larger and stronger (fast-twitch) muscle fibers occurs. Thus, when the load increases from light to heavy, there is a progressive increase in the number of muscle fibers involved in the contraction.[1] In essence, light loads, regardless of how many sets and reps you perform with them, recruit primarily slow-twitch muscle fibers, which have the lowest capacity to increase in size. Heavier loads recruit fast-twitch fibers in addition to the slow-twitch fibers already activated. From this we can conclude, quite without fear of contradiction, that the amount of weight lifted, as opposed to the speed of the contraction, is what recruits and stimulates the greatest amount of muscle fibers, thereby allowing for the greatest increases in size and strength.

As a result, you must consistently strive to lift heavier and heavier weights if so doing will increase your Power Factor. Consistent increases in size and strength are your goals, after all. If you have the fiber recruitment potential to bench-press 200 pounds for 6 sets of 30 repetitions, yet the most you ever lift in any given workout is 125 pounds for 6 sets of 30 repetitions, then neither your muscle mass nor your strength will ever increase. They don't have to; the muscles are only being called upon to do work that's well below their existing maximum capacity. (And that work, incidentally, is quite capable of being handled solely by the slow-twitch fibers, which happen to be the ones that have the least growth potential.)

HOW SIZE AND POWER ARE CREATED

What is the relationship between how a muscle grows and why a muscle grows? And please note that these are two very distinct issues, the answers to which are found in two distinct physiological processes. *How* muscle grows is through a process of overcompensation in direct proportion to the overload it has to contract against. The greater the overload imposed on the muscle, the greater the growth stimulation and, of course, the overcompensation (increase in muscle mass). *Why* muscle grows is because the body's muscular status quo (or homeostasis) has been threatened (via sufficient overload having been placed upon it) and because sufficient time has elapsed since that overload was imposed to allow the body's recuperative subsystems time to (1) recover from the stressor of training and (2) overcompensate or enlarge upon its existing stores of muscle mass to prevent a similar stressor from disrupting the body to the same extent the next time.

You can't acquire inordinate levels of power and muscle mass by gently coaxing or cajoling the muscles, nor by applying the popular though erroneous notion of "confusing" them. Instead, you must make them work to the limit of their uppermost capabilities for as long as possible, which (while individual variations may exist) is, for the vast majority, not really very long at all. Muscle growth is a systemic response to a tremendous overload having been imposed on the muscles via their contracting, whether concentrically, statically, eccentrically, or in combination, against a very heavy and demanding (high–Power Factor) resistance. If an individual is willing to exert himself maximally and uses progressive resistance in his workouts, the size and strength of his skeletal muscles will increase.

MUSCLE GROWTH AS SYSTEMIC, NOT LOCALIZED

Much of the confusion that has arisen in the realm of strength training has resulted from the belief that the muscle growth process is a localized rather than systemic phenomenon. This notion is erroneous, however. In fact, the central nervous system (CNS) triggers the growth process, a process that cannot be called into play by the isolated and protracted performance of highly repetitive tasks that are well within the body's existing muscular capacity. Growth is systemic, and the trigger mechanism that signals the body to grow can only be turned on by a call to arms from the CNS.

Growth isn't easy; it must literally be forced. Such being the case, how does one force growth with light weights or mild exertion? The answer is, One can't—at least not without steroids and growth drugs.

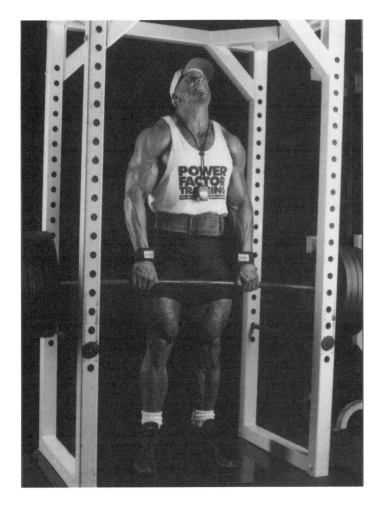

Muscle growth isn't easy. It must literally be forced.

RESEARCH ON REPETITION VARIATIONS

Heavy weights lifted as many times as possible within a given unit of time impose a maximum overload, not only on the localized muscles but, more importantly, on the CNS. This is the most important requirement for developing larger and stronger muscles. However, the Power

Index can actually decrease if the resistance is so heavy that only 1 or 2 repetitions are possible. In such cases, the actual muscular output (pounds lifted per minute) falls way off, thereby diminishing muscular overload.

Further, scientific research conducted by S. Grillner and M. Udo indicates that while parallel increases in load and muscle fiber recruitment occur, this process happens only up to a certain threshold point. They perceive that threshold to be at 50 percent of a muscle's maximum voluntary contractile ability. In fact, their research indicates that 90 percent of all available muscle fibers in a targeted muscle group have been activated with a load that is roughly 50 percent of a muscle's one-rep maximum.[2]

In other words, the weights selected for training should be heavy enough to recruit most of the available muscle fibers (slow, intermediate, and fast-twitch). But once this threshold is reached, going heavier will not necessarily recruit more muscle fibers. Depending upon innate fiber type distribution, it can actually diminish muscular output (your Power Factor).

ALTERATIONS IN NERVE DISCHARGE

It would appear that gains in strength obtained from a program utilizing weights in the range of 90 to 100 percent of a subject's one-rep maximum weight for low (1–6) repetitions are not necessarily the result of a still greater degree of fiber recruitment. Instead, the strength gains may result from alterations in the pattern of nerve discharge. Research by H. S. Milner-Brown and colleagues strongly corroborates this notion and goes on to reveal that the discharge of impulses appears to synchronize in response to muscular contraction against resistances close to 100 percent of a muscle's maximum voluntary contractile ability.[3]

Evidently, what happens in this respect is that the synchronization parlays into better timing between the nerves innervating the muscle and the rate of contraction. This results in the impulses for muscular contraction occurring more or less simultaneously, which heightens the electrical input into the muscle at one time and significantly amplifies the contractile force capacity of the existing fibers, irrespective of their actual size.

Therefore, the best results come from performing as many repetitions as possible using weights that are over 50 percent but under 100 percent of a trainee's one-rep maximum weight. (This broad range must exist owing to such diverse innate physiological conditions as predominant fiber type, neuromuscular contractile efficiency, age, and sex, as well as numerous other considerations among individuals.) The heavy weights will ensure that all available muscle fibers (slow, intermediate, and fast-twitch) will have been activated, while the higher repetitions will lead to greater muscular output as measured in pounds per minute (that is, overload). The result is the highest possible Power Index and greater muscle growth stimulation. All of this efficiency occurs maximally at the sweet spot (referred to in Chapter 2), where the weight on the bar and the number of corresponding reps generate your maximum Power Factor.

COMPETITIVE WEIGHTLIFTERS NEED HEAVIER WEIGHTS

For those more interested in the development of strength qua strength, it would obviously be of benefit to train with weights closer to 100 percent of their one-rep maximum (requiring lower repetitions), as so doing would improve their neural activity and, hence, their chances for competitive success. This has been corroborated by research conducted by D. H. Clarke, which indicates that such a systemic response to training can be elicited only when trainees employ weights approaching 90–100 percent of their one-rep maximum for sets of 1 to 6 repetitions.[4] In fact, anything less than this percentage would compromise their objectives of stimulating maximum strength increases. There would exist no need to improve upon or alter the existing patterns of nerve discharge within particular muscle groups during the performance of specific competitive lifts.

With all of the conclusions that have been predicated upon research emphasizing the percentage of one-rep maximum, it's important to keep in mind that, owing to the immense range of genetic variability among individuals, a one-size-fits-all repetition prescription is not only impractical but speculative at best. The bottom line in all of this is muscular output or overload. As long as an individual's Power Factor and Power Index are increasing consistently, the trainee is doing all that he reasonably can to stimulate maximum increases in his size and strength.

WHY MULTIPLE EXERCISES ARE NOT NECESSARY

Many bodybuilders have adopted the age-old contention that a variety of exercises for a particular muscle must be performed in order to activate all of a given muscle's fibers. However, as we've just learned, the law of muscle fiber recruitment renders this belief invalid. It's the force required to lift a weight that determines and activates the amount of fibers recruited, not the number of exercises performed. Choosing light-weight, multiple exercises is both inefficient and ineffective.

TRAINING FOR "SHAPE"

There's also a popular though erroneous belief (which exists in quite a few training circles) that by varying the angle at which a muscle is trained, the trainee will somehow be able to direct the stress imposed to specific areas of a muscle and can thereby "shape" the muscle being trained. This belief has absolutely no basis in fact. The reason is the way a muscle is innervated. The nerves that enter a given muscle divide out into threads that resemble branches on a tree. Each branch ends at the muscle cell and carries the electrochemical current that causes each muscle cell to contract. When this current is released, all of the cells serviced by the branch (a single neuron) contract simultaneously (the all-or-none law of muscle fiber contraction), not some to the exclusion of others. It's simply not possible to isolate one portion, border, or ridge of a muscle.

According to Dr. Fred Hatfield in his book *Bodybuilding: A Scientific Approach*, "the cells associated with each motor unit are spread all through the gross muscle; all portions of the gross muscle are affected similarly by a given exercise and therefore develop similarly. This is called the principle of noncontiguous innervation. Using many variations of an exercise for one muscle in no way ensures more growth or different growth patterning than does performing the basic exercise. . . . The shape of that muscle will not be affected by variations in the angle or position of stress application. Does this mean that all a bodybuilder has to do is perform the basic movement, and rid himself or herself of the array of supplemental exercises for a given muscle? I suspect it does."[5]

Muscle shape is a function of genetics. That's why the "muscle shaping" advocates can't perform an exercise to make a biceps muscle look like a triangle, a hexagon, or

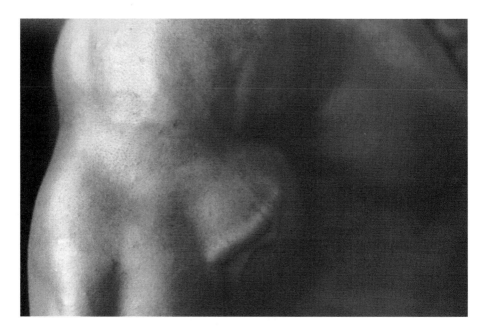

Muscle shape is a function of genetics. That's why the "muscle shaping" advocates can't perform an exercise to make a biceps muscle look like a triangle, a hexagon, or Mount Rushmore.

Mount Rushmore. Looking at it another way, suppose a sixteen-year-old had a crystal ball into which he could look to see what his muscles would look like when he is a maximally muscular twenty-one-year-old. He would see much larger, bulging muscles, but the look and shape of them would be as preordained as the shape of his nose or ears. He could train any way he wanted over the next five years, but his muscles would end up looking exactly like the ones in the crystal ball. There is no other choice. He could train with one set, ten sets, full range, strong range, isolation movements, compound movements, rock lifting, weight lifting, etc. But when he was at his maximum muscularity, his muscles would look the way they were programmed to look when his father's sperm hit his mother's egg.

So don't waste your time trying to shape a muscle into something it cannot become. All you can do is make your muscle smaller (through lack of use), larger (through progressive intensity), or stay the same (through no change in intensity).

OTHER ELEMENTS OF PRODUCTIVE EXERCISE

As important as it is to lift progressively heavier and heavier weights to stimulate continuous increases in size and strength, it's not the only factor. The bottom line is contraction. To induce maximum levels of muscle growth, as many of a muscle's fibers as possible must be made to contract simultaneously. The law of muscle fiber recruitment makes it abundantly clear that you must use a load of at least a threshold poundage, since in the body's ongoing effort to conserve energy, it activates only the minimum number of muscle fibers required to perform a particular movement for any given demand.

THE ROLE OF SUPPLY AND DEMAND

As you can see, the relationship between muscular stimulation and growth is one of supply and demand. For muscle growth to be supplied, there must first have been a very serious demand for it. After all, the primary concern of all living organisms is the acquisition and preservation of energy in order to better maintain the body's internal status quo, known as homeostasis. The growth of muscle tissue beyond normal levels is, in fact, a disruption of this status quo and requires additional energy for building and maintenance. Muscles will grow only when there is a tremendous physiological demand for them to do so. If a muscle's existing level of size and strength is adequate for handling workloads normally encountered (normal Power Factors), there will be no growth. There is no need for it.

The growth of muscle tissue, then, is a process that must literally be forced to take place. What is important to keep in mind is the fact that the human body will do everything it possibly can to maintain its existing condition. It will not waste precious resources building a larger musculature than it perceives to be necessary. It's up to you to give your body a reason to grow progressively larger and stronger muscles.

This can only be accomplished through maximum muscular output training and heavy weights. Power Factor Training, utilizing the enlightened technique of strongest-range repetitions, has been shown to deliver the greatest possible amount of overload to a working muscle. This, in turn, stimulates the body's overcompensation mechanism into action and results very quickly in maximal increases in the size and strength of its muscle tissue.

A STRONGER MUSCLE IS A BIGGER MUSCLE

It's a physiological fact that a muscle's strength is directly proportional to its cross-sectional area. In other words, if you want to get bigger, you've got to get stronger, and vice versa. The major physiological response to overload training is an increase in muscle fiber size. Trained muscle fibers tend to be larger than untrained muscle fibers. However, a variety of factors affect muscle strength and size. The type and density of muscle fibers, the location of tendon insertions, and the length of muscle bellies are inherited characteristics that cannot be altered through training. Consequently, some people possess a greater genetic potential for developing muscle size and strength.

It's not always possible to assess muscle strength solely by external measurements. Because greater muscle strength is accompanied by greater muscle weight, body composition evaluations provide a better means for determining changes in an individual's muscle mass. Although not everyone can develop huge muscles, everyone can

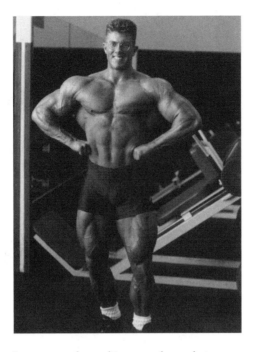

Stronger muscles are bigger muscles, and vice versa.

increase muscle density and strength through Power Factor Training.

NOTES

1. Research conducted by H. S. Milner-Brown and colleagues empirically validated the fact that the load imposed upon muscle during contraction is the major factor dictating the type and volume of muscle fiber recruitment. The results of their research were published in *Journal of Physiology*, 230, 359 (1973).
2. S. Grillner and M. Udo, *Acta Physiol. Scand.*, 81, 571 (1971).
3. H. S. Milner-Brown et al., *J. Physiol.*, 230, 385 (1973).
4. D. H. Clarke, Adaptations in strength and muscular endurance resulting from exercise, *Exercise & Sport Sciences Rev.*, 1, 73–102 (1973).
5. Dr. Fred Hatfield, *Bodybuilding: A Scientific Approach* (Chicago: Contemporary Books, 1988), 34.

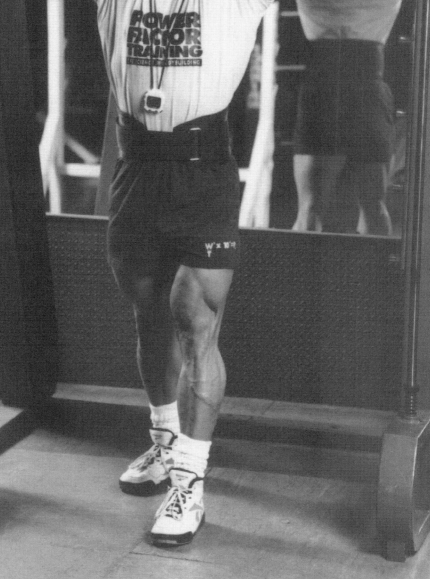

6

Developing Ligament Strength: The Key to Fantastic Power

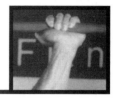

A ligament is a band of tissue, usually white and fibrous, that serves to connect bones at the body joints. Tendons, in contrast, are the tie or bond between muscles and the skeletal frame. Without question, you need strong ligaments to develop great strength. And, as mentioned, you need great strength to develop massive muscles.

The general public and many athletes have the idea that a man with large muscles must be strong, and all things being equal, this is correct. However, it's true only if the muscles have been developed through resistance exercise where poundages have increased gradually over a period of time, so enlarging the muscles' size and strength to make them equal to the demands put upon them. Consequently, a man with large but improperly trained muscles need not be strong at all. But one with rugged ligament structure invariably displays great natural power.

THE ACQUISITION OF SUPER POWER

While it's important to develop strong ligaments and tendons in order to support and lift heavy weights and, of course, to provide strong attachments for muscles undergoing intense contractions, tendons don't contract or otherwise aid in the lifting of the weight; only muscles do that. Even so, the tendons transmit the forces to the bones and move them.

The heavy partial movements that you perform during Power Factor Training not only develop and stimulate tremendous muscular growth, they develop and strengthen the ligaments, tendons, and even the bones to a certain degree. In other words, to develop maximum strength in your tendons and ligaments, you have to gain muscular strength. The two march in lockstep. The difference between mediocre and colossal strength lies in the pulling power of the ligaments working in conjunction with their accompanying muscles.

Bodybuilders who pump up their arms through daily workouts of light-weight, low-intensity activity don't enjoy the corresponding rise in strength and musculature that an increase in resistance would have caused. Only when greater muscle mass comes as a result of greater efforts (the handling of heavier and heavier weights) can ligament toughening really take place and fantastic strength result.

The legendary bodybuilder and strength athlete John Grimek is certainly the embodiment of what strong ligament strength can produce. Grimek built his tremendous muscle mass almost exclusively by using the aforementioned principle and techniques such as partial repetitions. Grimek told us that the most valuable piece of training advice ever given him was that offered by the late Canadian strength pioneer George Jowett. According to Grimek,

> *Jowett told me, "The best way to get strength is to support a lot of weight in certain positions. More than you can lift normally. . . . This will strengthen your ligaments, your tendons, and you get more strength out of that than you would if you were just doing flexing exercises." Which was true, as I found out, because you're subjecting your muscles to more stress and more weight than you've ever lifted prior to that, and it really worked well for me. . . . I got up to supporting overhead just over 1,000 pounds.*

Looking at the joints of legendary strong men such as Kazmaier and Grimek, people are compelled to comment not only on the size of their musculature, but also on their very pronounced tendons, which appear to have been forged of the strongest steel. The tendons of these men speak volumes for the power their muscles are carrying. Conversely, less-developed ligaments and tendons almost invariably mean weaker muscles, especially in the region of the legs. When an athlete starts to show signs of slowing down, it's sometimes said that he's becoming "weak in the knees." In fact, the knee is the joint that tends to buckle first under heavy weight. Leg strength depends heavily on ligaments and tendons.

To build power in the knee and hip joints—specifically within ligaments and tendons—you can't beat partial repetitions utilizing a range of only three to four inches. Movements such as the leg press are particularly effective in this regard and also quite safe, owing to the built-in safety factor of the safety pins, which prevent an accident should you descend too low. Really monstrous poundages can be handled in this exercise for multiple repetitions, a combination that promotes very rapid gains in both size and strength. Training with conventional methods, the athlete cannot lift enough weight with his hands or legs alone to maximally tax the muscles of either region, which results in reduced muscular development.

BODY STRUCTURE AND YOUR POTENTIAL FOR POWER

If you can visualize your body as a building, you'll get a better idea of the importance of its connective tissue. Like any structure, the human body is closely knit and of many parts. The muscles serve to move the joints and keep the body upright and in balance. The muscles are composed of microscopic bundles of tissue, bound together or enclosed by a white substance known as fascia. It is this connective tissue that gives the muscles their tensile strength. The muscle mass is enclosed on the outside in a strong sheath of this fascia. At the end of the muscle mass, the fascia become a tendon, itself attached to other connective tissue or bones. Every internal organ is covered with connective tissue, and its strength determines the quality or standard of performance of any athlete, for it is this tissue that is usually injured in athletic accidents.

Obviously, then, the more effort the bodybuilder or weightlifter takes to make this connective tissue stronger, the more powerful the muscles are going to be, especially in movements and positions that require strength to support or handle extremely heavy poundages. The more powerful the tendons and ligaments become, the less risk there is of suffering any severe muscle strain, tear, or other ligament or tendon injuries. Developing stronger ligaments, tendons, and joints through Power Factor Training opens the door to strength gains beyond the realm of most athletes' wildest expectations.

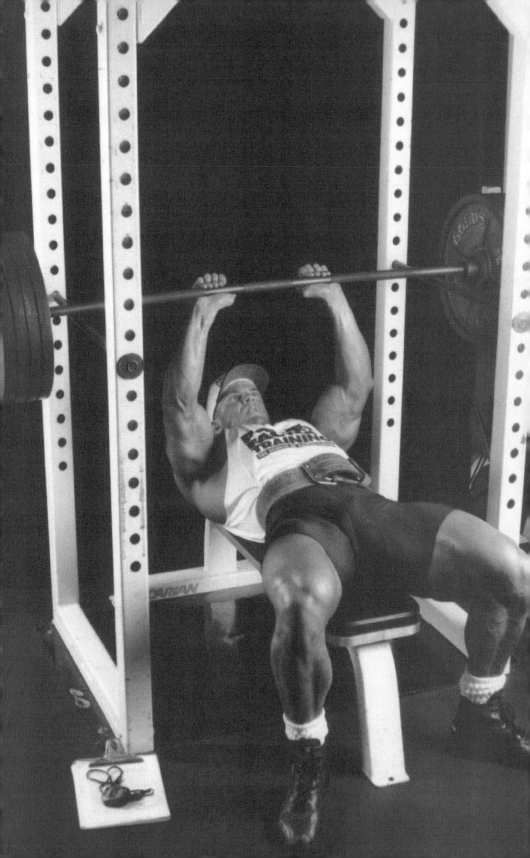

7

Strong-Range Partials: Why They're So Effective

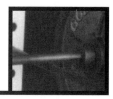

Anybody who's been involved in bodybuilding for any length of time will tell you that nothing builds thick, powerful pectorals like the bench press and that no other exercise is quite as effective as the Olympic press for building massive, powerful shoulders. After all, they are among the most basic of bodybuilding exercises. However, it is also known that the greatest development of these muscles comes about only from using very heavy exercising poundages.

As a result, the perennial question posed in the quest for bigger, more powerful muscles is, How can I continually handle more weight? The answer is found in the technique of maximum-overload partials—partial repetitions performed in the muscle's strongest range of motion. These are the cornerstone of Power Factor Training.

Among strength athletes and weightlifters of renown, many have used the technique of partial repetitions.

SUCCESS STORIES: BUILDING STRENGTH

Among strength athletes and weight lifters of renown, many have used the technique of partial repetitions, but few, if any, have recognized the full significance of its potential. Nevertheless, when they employed the technique, all admitted that they knew they were on to something. Consider the following stories.

Paul Anderson, the famed Olympic gold medalist (1956) who hit upon the method of performing partial repetitions early in his career, became a world champion before the age of twenty-one. His back lift of 6,270 pounds still stands some forty years later, according to the *Guinness Book of Records,* as "the greatest weight ever lifted by a human being." Anderson was one of the pioneers in the field of partials, having made an in-depth study of the technique's effectiveness by incorporating it into his own workouts. Power Racks and Smith Machines did not exist in Anderson's time, so the mighty native of Toccoa, Georgia, would perform his partials by suspending massively loaded barbells from chains hanging off the branches of trees in his backyard. These weights would be lowered to a point that was roughly four inches above his head, and Anderson would practice his partial repetitions from this range.

In conversation with the authors, Anderson spoke highly of the effectiveness of the technique: "I've done them throughout the years. The first partial movement I did was the quarter squat. When I did them for a few weeks without doing full squats, I wanted to see what full squats would be like, so I started doing the full squats again, and the weight felt like a feather!"

Ronald Walker, the great English Olympic weight lifter, developed his strength through limited-range work to such a capacity that he could support more than 600 pounds overhead.

Anthony Clark, the first teenager in history to bench-press 612 pounds and the first man to reverse-grip bench 701 pounds, told the authors of his experience with the partial-reps principle:

> *I think they work! If you're doing heavy partials, that's providing a real overload, which causes a quick adaptation by the body. Once you go back down to a regular style of training with a lighter weight, it's much easier. I've used partials myself and, because of the length of the bar, you can only really go slightly over 1,000 pounds, which I'll do on movements like squats, and I'm around 800 pounds on the bench press.*

Bill Kazmaier, whose numerous powerlifting championships and strong man titles earned him the additional title of being the "World's Greatest Strong Man," told the authors his thoughts about this great training technique: "I liked partials because of the overload they delivered. I did partial squats just to be able to handle the weight and also partial dead lifts to increase parts of the lockout. I did 1,000 pounds for partials in the squat as an assistance exercise, and . . . they were very helpful in adding muscle mass."

SUCCESS STORIES: BUILDING MUSCLE MASS

Partial repetitions, performed in the strongest range of motion, will do the same wondrous things for the bodybuilder seeking increased muscle mass as they have done for champion lifters in search of greater overall body power. Partials build amazing ligament, tendon, and muscle strength, which permits the bodybuilder to perform phenomenally heavy bench presses, military presses,

presses behind neck, and a host of other power movements that build tremendous whole-body power and very impressive muscular development. Here are five examples of how partial reps have stimulated not only phenomenal power development, but also tremendous increases in muscle mass.

John Grimek, a legendary bodybuilder and one of weight lifting's immortals as well, spoke to us about his experience in using partials to build not only colossal strength (he was able to support overhead a 1,000-pound weight slung from rafters on chains when he weighed only 185 pounds!) but also to develop his incredible muscle mass:

> I had rafters in my attic to which I hooked up some support straps where a bar would be suspended from these rafters and loaded up with weights. You see, the straps would support the barbell at a height that was about eye level so that you could perform movements like partial presses overhead and so forth. I could really make my exercises very heavy this way. I recall that they worked quite well. In fact, I got quite strong using these, at least for my size and age and so forth. I was much stronger than anybody around at the time. It really increased my power and muscle mass quite a bit.

Mike Mentzer, the first bodybuilder to successfully apply the discipline of science to his training and also, not accidentally, the first to ever garner a perfect score of 300 in competition (when he won the 1978 Mr. Universe contest in Acapulco, Mexico), was also a strong advocate of performing partial repetitions in his training. Regarding his experience with partials, Mentzer had this to say to his audience in *Muscle & Fitness* magazine:

> *The last time I engaged in any serious Power Rack work was when Casey Viator first moved to California in the late 1970s. . . . In the quarter squat Casey and I both got up to more than 1,100 pounds for a few reps. . . . We used 625 pounds for quarter reps in the incline press. . . . We both used similarly impressive poundages in the Dead Lift and Press Behind Neck. And while no one has ever accused either Casey or me of lacking size, we both noticed appreciable mass increases during that period of Power Rack work.*

When Mentzer and his brother, Ray, were performing partial-range Preacher curls for their biceps back in the late 1970s, he told us:

> *We would overload the bar for the Preacher curls from our usual 150 pounds for full-range reps to 220 pounds for partial reps. Using a Preacher bench perpendicular to the ground so the resistance didn't fall off in the top of the movement, one of us would lower the 220-pound bar to the halfway position, where the other's hands would stop the bar and possibly even give a slight boost to get the mammoth weight started back upward. Once the weight began its ascent, no assistance was given. About 4 reps performed in this all-out fashion were all we could take. After a set performed in said manner we'd immediately sit down to avoid falling down!*

Lou Ferrigno, the star of *The Incredible Hulk* television series and (at 6'5" and 320 pounds) also one of the most massive bodybuilders of all time, is another champion who utilizes the Power Factor technique of partial repetitions in his training, working up to 2,300 pounds on

partial leg presses! Ferrigno had this to say about his experience with partials:

> I used to do leg presses utilizing a full range of
> motion, going all the way down to the point where
> my knees would touch my upper chest on every rep
> of every set. After a few sets of this, my lower
> back would be killing me, but my thighs would
> have no pump at all. Eventually I started bending
> my knees just a bit and my thighs just went
> WHAM! My upper thighs blew right up!
> Eventually, they got up to 32 inches around!

Paul DeMayo, who is also known as "Quadzilla"
because of his astounding quadriceps development, is perhaps the brightest up-and-coming bodybuilder in the
sport today. Not surprisingly, he too has been a longtime
booster of partial repetitions:

> I don't believe in full reps. They're not for me at
> all. I do partials on calves, shoulders, and chest.
> Anytime I do a full-range rep on, say, calf raises,
> the stress comes off of my calves and onto my
> lower back and rear end. I used to train that way,
> thinking that was the correct way, and then one
> day I thought to myself, "Why don't I just shut my
> eyes, concentrate, and see at what point the ten-
> sion comes off my calves during the range of
> motion and at what point it's at its maximum?"
> For me, anything beyond a partial rep, and I don't
> get anything out of it. Keeping that in mind, now
> when I train my calves, I always use a half or par-
> tial rep—and my calves have grown!

Dorian Yates, at an off-season bodyweight of
295 pounds at 6 percent bodyfat, is easily the most massive Mr. Olympia champion in the history of bodybuild-

ing. Utilizing every high-intensity technique in the book, Dorian also employs the technique of partial reps when looking to up his training intensity dramatically to stimulate further muscle growth in the off-season:

> *Partials are something I've done with various exercises over the years in lieu of forced reps. Let's face it, in some exercises, it's just not practical to have forced reps. I know that on a barbell row, for example, I'll go to failure with full-range reps and then continue beyond failure with half and quarter reps until I can't even move the bar!*
>
> *Every year I train, I try to become smarter about finding better ways to increase my intensity. After all, at my level of development there comes a point of diminishing returns; I have to fight like hell for even a little bit more muscle growth. My body has basically become accustomed to things like training with straight sets, or some such way to extend my sets and make them ever harder, so I'm always looking for things like rest/pause or maximum negatives or some such things.*
>
> *I used some partials while preparing for the 1993 Mr. Olympia and found them to be very good. My way of using them was to perform them at the end of a set of regular-range repetitions on exercises such as incline barbell or machine presses and leg presses. I found that, when you fail doing positive reps, you still have some static or holding strength. And when you fail at static strength, you've still got some negative strength. And when you fail at that, you could probably still do partials. If the muscle can still function, then why not take it all the way?*

As you can see, partials allow you to lift much heavier weights than you would normally. Of course, the heavier the weights you lift, the greater the overload you're imposing on the muscles, which is the prime requisite for building massive muscles. You've got to train heavy to get big, and partials allow you to train in the heaviest possible manner.

THE POWER FACTOR LOOK

"It is a shame for a man to grow old without seeing the beauty and strength of which his body is capable."—Socrates

Power Factor Training, in addition to building stronger ligament and tendon strength, gives the body a very powerful, rugged look. You see this extraordinarily rugged look in the physiques of the athletes whose statements you've just read, as well as in the physiques of other athletes of today who train with very heavy poundages. People like Dorian Yates, Flex Wheeler, and John Sherman have the look. It's a look that more and more bodybuilders seem anxious to acquire.

Although you may never be able to lift weights as heavy as, say, John Grimek did, by lifting as much as you can and by making a concerted effort to increase your Power Factor on a per workout basis, you'll certainly develop your physique to its most muscularly massive limit. As you will see, Power Factor Training utilizing the technique of partial repetitions is the only system that can enable you to overcome the leverage and developmental deficiencies that nature may have foisted upon you. Give it a try for yourself, and watch your personal size and strength records skyrocket!

THE "WEAK LINK" ANALOGY

There is a popular maxim in strength training: A chain is only as strong as its weakest link. In other words, you're

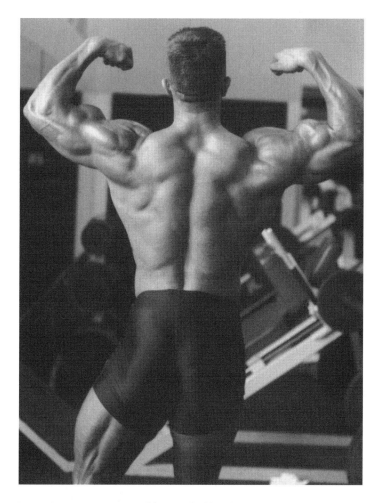

Power Factor Training, in addition to building ligament and tendon strength, gives the body a very powerful, rugged look.

only as strong in an exercise as you are in the weakest part of its range of motion (also known as the sticking point). This maxim, however, fails to take into account the fact that you have a choice in the matter; you don't have to train in your weakest range of motion.

With full-range repetitions, you're restricted to how much overload you can impose on your muscles due to the leverage deficiency, even though your muscles are capable of handling, in most cases, hundreds more pounds in the strongest range of the movement than you're presently subjecting them to. If your muscles are capable of lifting 500 pounds for 20 repetitions, yet the most you ever work out with is 150 for the same amount of reps, what reason has your body to alter its present muscle size? Obviously none, even if you "progress" by adding 1 or 2 repetitions or even 10 pounds to the exercise. The reason is that the level of muscular output is still well below what you're capable of.

If you remain locked into the notion that you must perform full-range movements (usually because that's the way "everybody else" performs them), maximum gains in the form of rapid increases in strength and muscle mass will never be forthcoming. Instead, you must think in terms of what your muscles are capable of handling in their strongest range of motion, not their weakest one. If you remain in the weak mode, then you'll only progress as quickly as your weakest link does, which is exasperatingly slow at best.

STRENGTH, FLEXIBILITY, AND ENDURANCE

The three benchmarks of physical fitness are strength, flexibility, and endurance. Power Factor Training is designed to accomplish one and only one of these objectives: strength. Although you can improve flexibility by performing some full-range weight-lifting exercises or stimulate the cardiovascular system (to improve endurance) by performing high repetitions with heavy partial movements, such techniques would be vastly inferior to yoga and running or other specific stretching and endurance exercises. To develop cardiovascular endurance, weight lifting could garner some improvement but will never equal cross-country skiing, distance running, or other more specific exercises. But for developing strength, nothing can deliver better results than weight lifting, and no method allows you to lift more weight than Power Factor Training.

POLEMICS FROM THE TRADITIONALISTS

Somewhere along the line, you can expect to hear the disparaging statement, With partials you're not really as strong as you appear on paper because you're not doing a full-range rep. This is an argument advanced only by people who enjoy arguing. In reality, it's an argument that has no end. For example, cambered bench press bars that force your hands below chest level allow you to achieve a greater range of motion than a straight Olympic barbell is capable of providing. But does this fact mean that all powerlifters are weak or "not really as strong as they appear on paper" because their range of motion is less with a straight Olympic bar than it is with a cambered bar?

The truth of the matter is that your body doesn't have a clue as to whether you're performing a full-range rep. All it knows is that your muscles are being called upon to lift a very heavy weight for a lot of repetitions, which requires a tremendous amount of energy to accomplish. More muscle fibers have to be activated as force requirements (the effort required to move heavy resistance) dictate fiber involvement, more hormones have to be secreted, more blood has to be sent to the working muscles at a faster rate, waste products have to be cleared, and the initiation of the Krebs cycle and a host of other metabolic activities have to take place. The body isn't as concerned about such aesthetic conditions as whether your muscles are performing full-range repetitions. In fact, in terms of its energy systems, the body can't tell if you're training your quads or your pecs; its sole concern is how much energy and fiber recruitment are required to get the job done. And, obviously, with strongest-range training, the greater weight (overload) employed necessitates greater energy production in terms of what's necessary to fuel the increased fiber recruitment and muscular output—which, as the clinical studies cited earlier empirically demonstrated, is the only stimulus that induces muscle growth. The bottom line is that with strongest-range training, your muscles are made to contract against the heaviest weights possible, and that is exactly what's required to stimulate maximum muscle growth.

FUNCTIONAL STRENGTH

It should be obvious by now that with Power Factor Training, you're not engaging in a stretching competition. You're training for the express purpose of developing your absolute maximum muscular mass and strength, nothing more. Training the muscles in their strongest range of motion develops what is termed functional strength, as doing so builds tremendous and practical bodily power that is both utilized and necessary for all of your day-to-day activities and any emergencies that should crop up.

An illustration of the importance of functional strength occurs when you trip and fall. Your arms reflexively go out far in front of you to help cushion and absorb your descent. They do not first recoil to a point one or two inches from your chest. The reason why this doesn't happen is obvious; your arms are strongest when they're almost completely extended, and you're better able to absorb many times your bodyweight from such a position. Likewise, if you push a car out of a ditch or down a road, you do so with your arms almost fully extended. When your legs assist in the movement, you certainly don't make it a point to touch your glutes to your heels with every step in order to achieve a full range of motion. Doing so would be both unnecessary and impractical in the attempt to generate maximum power quickly.

You can readily see how this principle could easily be applied to most sports as well. Have you ever seen a football lineman prepare to blitz through the line to the intended target by first squatting down until his haunches are resting on the backs of his calves and drawing his elbows back so far that his hands are at the outside of his chest? Of course not! To do so would represent a sacrifice of strength, movement, speed, and energy on his part. Functional strength for a football player resides in a movement of between four and five inches. This is the range where he'll build all the explosive strength necessary for his legs and arms to move from a semi-extended to a fully extended position in the shortest possible time. In other words, training for functional strength via short-range, quick, and explosive movements will have the player at his intended target as quickly as possible, and when he arrives there, he'll be completely prepared to do his job in his strongest functional range. This makes him less prone to injury and able to perform more effectively.

In contrast, full-range repetitions are useful only for performing in artificial games and contests, such as powerlifting. Unless a full-range bench press competition somehow becomes a crucial method for determining the outcome of a football game or bodybuilding contest, learning to become more efficient in the skill of full-range or "weak link" bench-pressing is entirely unnecessary. Your goal as a bodybuilder, strength athlete, or football player is to build strength and size, period. And, as discussed previously, full-range exercise simply makes this goal impossible to obtain, at least as far as your potential actually allows. In fact, not one study has ever been conducted that has proved that a full range of motion is an absolute requirement for stimulating maximum increases in size and strength.

Further, the range of motion required to tax your functional strength is the safest range of all, simply because you are at your strongest in that range. Injuries occur in the weakest range of motion when a load is imposed on muscles, ligaments, joints, and connective tissue that exceeds their structural integrity. Functional strength training means that you're not subjecting your muscles, tendons, and ligaments to exaggerated arcs of motion and/or injury, inducing leverages solely for the sake of performing a barbell movement over some arbitrary distance.

THE NATURAL RANGE

Outside of the gym, virtually no one uses a full range of motion. Partial reps are more in keeping with the natural range of motion that our muscles utilize on a day-to-day basis. They are the safest types of repetitions to perform, and—more to the point—they produce fantastic results. A sprinter, for example, can develop his or her legs quite well simply by running, which is patently a partial-range exercise. Again, we can't stress too strongly that nowhere has it been empirically established that performing exercises over an exaggerated, or "full range," of motion will stimulate more muscle fibers. The analogy of the sprinter should establish conclusively that you don't need to touch your butt to your heels (as, for example, when squatting) in order to stimulate size increases in your thighs. By locking yourself into the notion that you should utilize only full-range movements in your training, you'll only become as strong as your weakest link in the movement will allow. Your true maximum strength capacity, maximum fiber recruitment, and maximum size potential will be left almost completely untapped and unfulfilled.

Our bodies were not designed to lift weights according to the strict requirements of man-made games. Consequently, when you lift a weight by these artificial rules of range, you end up selling your muscles short in developing maximum size and strength. Your muscles are capable of doing almost any job you require of them, but exaggerations of form or full-range rules may prevent them from doing the weight-lifting job of which they are capable and may even cause injury.

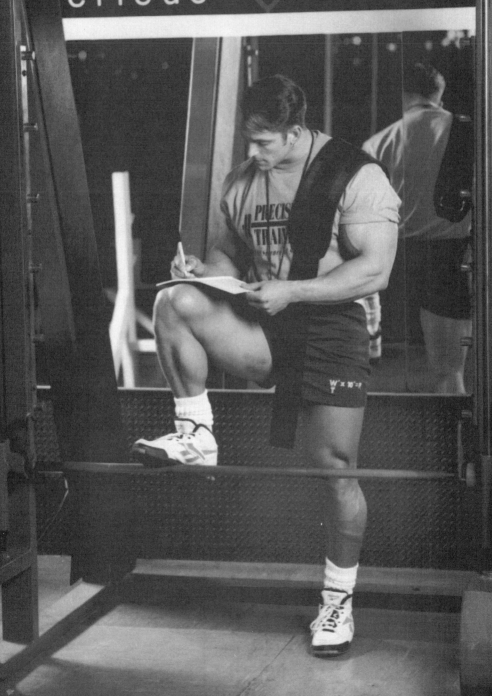

8

Your Ideal Routine

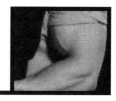

Just what is the "ideal" training routine? How many sets? How many reps? How many exercises per body part? And how many days per week should one train to stimulate maximum gains in size and strength? These are valid questions to be sure, but until recently nobody had an answer to them. There were opinions, but very few of these opinions were consistent, and fewer still had any scientific basis. When we looked into the realm of the requirements of productive exercise, we were surprised to find that the answers to these queries came forth rather readily, once we took time to analyze the cause-and-effect relationship between size and strength.

When we embarked on the development of Power Factor Training, we did so with no preconceived biases or prejudices of how to train. No "opinions" were granted legitimacy. Instead, we went by what science had revealed to be physiological facts, such as how our bodies react to stress; what exercises allow the use of the heaviest weights and, hence, yield the greatest pounds per minute of

What is the "ideal" training routine? How many sets, reps, and exercises per body part?

exercise (thereby allowing for the greatest amount of muscular output); what training methods deliver the greatest overload to the muscles; and how frequently such an overload can be applied to bring about a purely anabolic condition of the human body. These were our guidelines. Being facts, they were not subject to change but instead straightforward and even obvious. We had no interest in the dogmatic preservation of bodybuilding tradition (or any other tradition, for that matter). Our sole objective was purely to discover what was required in the way of progressive resistance exercise to produce the fastest possible increases in both muscular size and strength.

Once we viewed the issue in this context, no other considerations held any meaning. It was at once obvious that, in order to gain muscle mass, we had to stimulate muscle growth. For maximum possible gains, there had to be maximum growth stimulation. At this point, the question became, How is muscle stimulated? The answer came back, By imposing a progressive overload upon it. Another question then had to be asked: Which technique yields the greatest overload? The answer to both queries, we discovered, was the technique of strongest-range repetitions, wherein the greatest weight could be used to dramatically overload the muscles in a way that no other technique could even remotely approach. When the muscular overload in training is as high as possible, growth will have been stimulated and will occur as long as your training sessions don't occur too frequently.

The whole idea behind lifting weights is to generate high-intensity muscular overload. If you were to just flex your elbow up and down, with no weight in your hand, your biceps muscle would not increase in size or strength. We lift weights in order to increase the intensity of work and trigger growth. But how is that intensity measured? It isn't. For over 100 years of strength training, no system has ever quantified the amount of overload—until the Power Factor was innovated. Once a means of measuring overload is at hand, it becomes simple to quantify the value of every exercise and to guarantee that progress is taking place on a workout-to-workout basis.

YOUR TRAINING SCHEDULE

The first thing the body does immediately after a workout is to recoup the energy and reserves lost during the workout. The processes of recovery and growth are separate, each requiring a certain amount of time. While recovery of an individual muscle may be quite rapid, the recovery of the overall physical system (also known as systemic recovery) was typically thought to require anywhere from forty-eight to seventy-two hours. However, recent research, backed up by the authors' personal experience, would indicate that if the overload was of sufficient intensity to stimulate strength and size increases, systemic recovery may take anywhere from one to six weeks. During that time training would be both unnecessary and counterproductive, as it would make further inroads into the individual's limited recovery ability.

If you are operating blind (with no measure of your muscular output), you will have no way to discern accurately whether you have recovered from your previous workout. But if ever you reach a point where you're not progressing in Power Factor Training, your Power Factor and/or Power Index will reveal it instantly. This will help you schedule your workouts for maximum benefit.

Because you are stronger after each workout, your "ideal routine" changes every time. For example, we started our own Power Factor Training on a three-day-per-week split routine, training half the body (shoulders, traps, biceps, triceps) on one day and the other half (lats, pecs, lower back, legs, and calves) on the next training day on an alternating basis. We would train on Mondays, Wednesdays, and Fridays, allowing a full forty-eight hours (and an additional twenty-four hours on the weekends) to elapse between workouts so the processes of recovery and growth could occur. For the first month and a half, this spacing was perfect; our progress soared on a per workout basis. Soon an overhead press limit weight rose from a respectable 185 pounds to a monstrous 405 pounds. Likewise with bench presses; what had previously yielded 6 reps with 165 now was, 70 days later, giving way to 485 pounds for 20 reps. And the leg presses just flat out skyrocketed, from 800 for 6 to 1,325 for 35!

Obviously some major changes had occurred. After all, a weaker muscle (such as ours were when we started training) contracting maximally requires less metabolic fuel and produces different quantities of by-products and wastes than does a stronger muscle contracting maximally and moving a greater weight. The result was that we were now much stronger than when we began training, and our ability to generate maximum levels of overload had risen to such high levels that we were beginning to exceed our bodies' capacities to recover from our workouts. Our greater muscle mass (and we were gaining mass steadily), working at greater output levels, was using up much more fuel and producing much heavier quantities of waste products than we were even remotely capable of when we first started training. (As a side note, total oxygen uptake in a trained muscle working at maximum capacity has been shown to increase in some cases up to thirty times its original resting capacity!)

At this point, we began to experience a very strong disinclination to train on our scheduled three-day-a-week program. We evidently had been stimulating growth with every workout, but due to the increased overload and corresponding increased demand on our recovery abilities, we apparently were not allowing sufficient time for both the recovery and growth processes to take place. All of this was reflected in a plateau then a decrease in our Power Index numbers. The only logical conclusion was that we would have to reduce our training days per week.

At this point, we reduced our Power Factor Training sessions to only two days per week (Tuesdays and Fridays) and sometimes even once a week. The result? Our strength gains made another quantum leap upward! Our overhead presses were now being done with 475 pounds, our bench presses with 525 pounds for 20 reps, our repetition barbell shrugs with 600 pounds, and our leg presses went over the moon to 1,600 pounds for 20 reps!

VARYING RECOVERY APPLICATIONS

Power Factor Training's effect on the body is so dramatic that a prolonged recovery period is mandatory. The question at this point changes from How soon *can* I go back to the gym? to How soon *must* I go back to the gym? Some individuals may only require one high-intensity Power Factor Training session per week in order to stimulate an adaptive response from the body, depending on their innate adaptability to exercise. Others may require two weeks off between workouts for recovery and growth to manifest. Still others may require upwards of six weeks. What's becoming clear is that there exists a wide range of variation among individuals with regard to their personal recovery ability (that is, their ability to tolerate peak overload training). By closely monitoring your Power Factor and Power Index numbers, you can adjust the frequency of your workouts to ensure either steady increases in size and strength or simply maintenance of your maximum strength. Any steady decline of Power

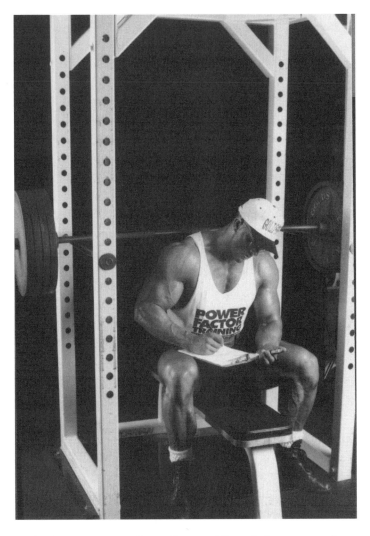

By closely monitoring your Power Factor and Power Index, you can adjust the frequency of your workouts in a manner that ensures either steady increases in size and strength or maintenance of your maximum strength.

Factor or Power Index numbers is an indicator of over-training.

One thing is for certain in this regard, however, and that is if you are training with maximum overload and if your workouts are both brief (less than one hour) and infrequent enough that you don't use up all of your recuperative reserves merely to compensate for the exhaustive effects of the workout itself, you will grow. The very fact that you grew stronger is proof that you fully recovered from your workout.

A WORD ABOUT REPETITIONS

Despite what some trainers will tell you, there is no magic number of reps to perform for building mass or increasing definition. Remember that muscular definition is primarily the result of losing subcutaneous fat so that the muscles directly beneath the skin appear in bold relief. To achieve this degree of definition, you really don't have to train with weights at all; running even a mile a day will burn far more calories from your body than would the performance of some extra sets of bench presses or cable crossovers.

In any event, it is well substantiated that training with peak overload causes the greatest adaptive response by the CNS. As long as you're training with your highest possible Power Factor and Power Index, you will have done all you reasonably can to stimulate an adaptive increase in your muscle mass stores. The sole focus of your training should be on what gives you higher numbers. The Power Factor and Power Index numbers are what is important, not whether or not you are doing 8 reps or 12 or 17 or 63.

While specific, one-size-fits-all repetition schemes normally apply to only a small cross section of the populace, it is of interest to note that research conducted back in 1956 by F. A. Hellebrandt and S. J. Houtz reported that when subjects engaged in lifting a weight that induced fatigue at 25 repetitions for up to 10 sets, it produced a very profound effect in muscle tissue. In fact, muscular output could increase by over 200 percent in as little as fifteen training sessions. Such progress fits perfectly in line with what we have experienced when performing partial repetitions using heavy weights with similar repetitions in Power Factor Training. According to Hellebrandt in his own conclusions, "The living machine operates under such wide margins of safety that it is difficult to deplete hidden reserves of power in short periods of exercise consisting of small numbers of contractions."[1]

Although there is much merit in Hellebrandt's conclusions, you should still experiment with various numbers of sets and reps to see what combination can give you your highest Power Factor and Power Index numbers, using the preceding guidelines. As long as you don't train too often (no more than three times a week), you'll grow bigger and stronger from workout to workout.

LIFTING HEAVY WEIGHTS SAFELY

One of the stated objections to training with heavy weights is that it's injurious to the bones and connective tissues. However, this objection is without merit. Training with heavy weights is actually quite safe as long as the emphasis is on lifting the weight, as opposed to attempting to thrust it or torque it. Trying to move a weight that's simply too heavy for the muscles involved requires the use of "outside" forces such as momentum and body leverage. Lifting a heavy weight with the aid of these outside forces amplifies the force transmitted to the joints and connective tissues, thereby increasing the risk of injury.

All exercises in Power Factor Training should be performed in strict form to eliminate the involvement of these outside forces. This is not to indicate that all your reps must be slow-motion affairs, however. Studies have indicated that more fibers are involved in utilizing a quicker rep cadence (at least on the concentric or lifting phase of the rep), providing that the muscle itself is responsible for the velocity of the resistance and that the overload is under the total control of the muscle at all times. Once the velocity exceeds muscular control, the chances of injury increase tremendously.

It is also advisable to obtain a good lifting belt that offers adequate support to your lumbar area for overhead lifts and other heavy exercises. In addition, we've found that wrist wraps and hooks are absolutely essential in movements such as dead lifts, pulldowns, and shrugs, as your muscular strength in the larger muscle groups will quickly surpass that of your smaller forearm muscles. When you are performing bench presses and overhead presses, strong wrist wraps are mandatory.

NOTE

1. F. A. Hellebrandt & S. J. Houtz, *Physical Therapy Review*, 36 (1956).

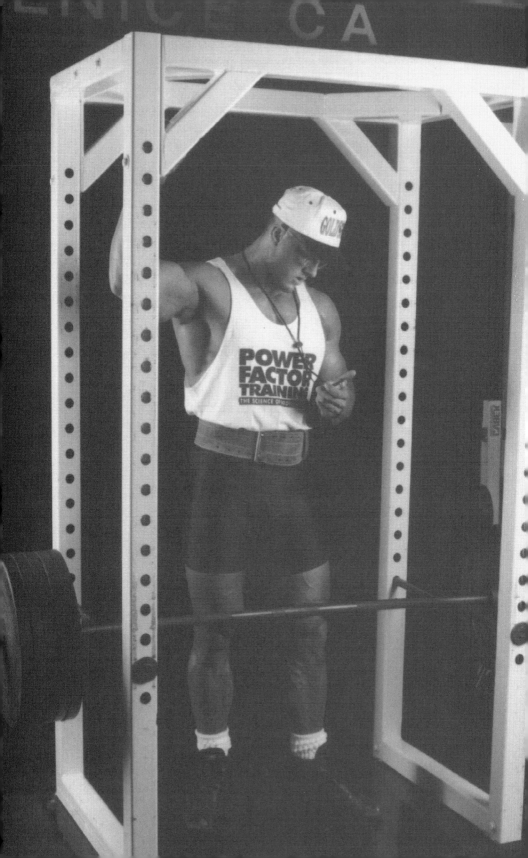

9

The Ten Best Exercises for Power Factor Training

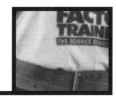

This chapter describes ten exercises that are well suited to Power Factor Training. These exercises all involve heavy compound movements that will tax a muscle or muscle group to its maximum ability. In short, these exercises require the highest Power Factor. When you first switch to strongest-range training, you will note that you can lift heavier weight and, because you lift it a shorter distance, more reps per unit of time.

Also, this type of training will require a few workouts in order to establish what you are actually capable of lifting with this new method. So do not be overly impressed with the first big increase in your numbers, as it is more likely due to your improved technique and your selection of more appropriate weights as you adjust.

Important Note: To perform strong-range exercises safely, it is *mandatory* to use either a Power Rack or a Smith Machine in order to physically limit the range of motion. By definition, strong-range

To perform strong-range exercises safely, it is mandatory to use either a Power Rack (pictured) or a Smith Machine in order to physically limit the range of motion of the weight.

training involves lifting weights that you are incapable of lifting in your weak range. Consequently, if the weight should be permitted to descend into your weak range, you will be powerless to move it and could suffer great injury. Use a Power Rack or Smith Machine, or do not perform these exercises.

THE WORKOUT

Frequency: One of the most important things to remember is that using a fixed training frequency with progressive overload training will lead to eventual stagnation in 100 percent of cases. It's a metabolic law. You can begin this program on a three-day-a-week schedule of, for example, Monday, Wednesday, and Friday, but don't expect to keep that schedule for more than three or four weeks. Soon (as dictated by your numbers) you will need to train on, say, Monday and Thursday only. Next you will need to adjust it to Mondays only and finally to workouts that are eight, ten, twelve, or more days apart. This is the *only* way to ensure consistent progress on a workout-to-workout basis.

Rotation: Perform Workouts A and B on alternate workout days. For example, during Week 1, do A on Monday, B on Wednesday, and A on Friday. During Week 2, do B on Monday, A on Wednesday, and B on Friday. Never perform the same workout twice in a row.

Rest Periods: Ninety percent of trainees require a rest of 15 to 90 seconds between sets of an exercise. However, we do not specify an exact rest time because it is so variable among trainees. Take the time you need to catch your breath and get some of the lactic acid out of your muscles, but don't waste time—the clock is ticking.

Rep Speed: By definition, the speed of reps using partials is much quicker than for full-range movements. Your cadence will be comparatively fast. As a result your sets will also contain more reps (20, 30, 40, or possibly more per set).

Reps and Sets: Begin this program by performing 2 sets of 20 reps for each exercise. This will permit you to gauge the correct weights to use and number of reps to perform. However, to ensure increases in overload, you should adjust your sets, reps, and weights as your training progresses.

Beginning Weights: Whether you realize it or not, you are already capable of lifting weights in strongest-range training that are far heavier than you use in conventional training. However, as a starting point you should use 70 to 90 percent of your maximum full-range weight when beginning this program. The fact is, where you begin is really not very important, since you will very soon be engineering workouts that will tax your maximum strength. Look upon the first three or four workouts as a learning process that helps you zero in on your sweet spot and maximum strongest-range output.

Timekeeping: Time your individual exercises with a stopwatch so that you have exact times for each exercise. Time your entire workout with the clock on the wall. During an exercise keep the stopwatch running even when you are getting a drink of water, reading the gym bulletin board, or answering the phone. But in no event should you include the time you spend warming up in your exercise time. Doing so provides an incentive to increase weights for warm-ups and essentially turns your warm-up into part of your workout, so don't do it.

Consistency is the key to having meaningful comparisons. For example, if you always perform two light sets to warm up just before bench presses, then that time will always be included in your overall time (the clock on the wall). But since it's the same amount of time every workout, it just factors out of comparisons. The rule is, Keep time the same way every workout.

Warm-up: The warm-up you use is up to your judgment. We cannot specify a one-size-fits-all warm-up, as there are so many human variables (age, past injuries, innate flexibility, etc.) and even environmental ones like the gym temperature. You may warm up entirely before a workout or just warm up individual muscles and joints before each exercise. You are the judge of when you have warmed up adequately to begin your workout.

Range of Motion: The more we learn about the role of range of motion in stimulating new muscle growth, the more we realize its lack of importance. As it stands, it is safe to say that the range of motion that you move a weight has an importance somewhere between very little and none. The first edition of *Power Factor Training* counseled ranges that were about double and in some cases triple what we are now recommending. The actual experience of thousands of trainees has proved that ranges can be greatly reduced with improved, not diminished, results. In fact, the authors recently conducted a study in which subjects used zero range of motion (static holds) and stimulated very substantial new muscle growth. So don't be tempted to increase the ranges of motion because you feel guilty for "cheating." Let the other guys feel guilty for wasting time and motion.

WORKOUT A

Standing Barbell Press

The first exercise you'll be performing in Workout A is standing barbell presses performed in either a Power Rack or, preferably, a Smith Machine. The standing barbell press is a movement that will build extremely powerful muscles in your deltoids, traps, and upper back.

The Power Factor Training method of performing this exercise is as follows:

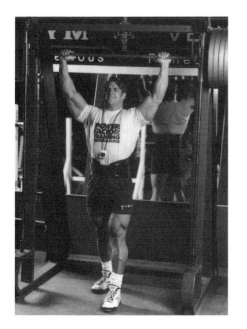
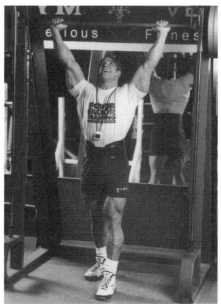

Standing barbell press—start position   *Standing barbell press—finish position*

1. Adjust the height of your support (whether in a Power Rack or on a Smith Machine) so that the bar is about two to four inches below the height of a fully extended rep. As soon as you develop a feel for the movement and are able to hoist some appreciable poundages, shorten up on your range with a two-inch maximum in the distance the bar travels.

2. From a standing position, with your hands approximately three inches wider on each side than your shoulders, press the bar upward until your elbows are locked.

3. Lower the bar slightly, just enough to break the lock in your elbows, and simultaneously dip your legs in a simulated split position (one knee just slightly forward and unlocked while the back leg remains slightly bent as well).

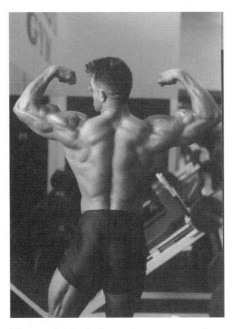

The standing barbell press is a movement that will build extremely powerful muscles in your deltoids, traps, and upper back.

4. From this lower position, push/press the weight to the fully extended position, using some slight assistance from your calves and quads. This is really just a slight dipping movement, designed to assist you pressing that heavy weight upward.

It is important to get a good, quick cadence going with your reps, in order to increase your work output in a unit of time, so don't be afraid to bang them out fast until you've reached 15 to 20 repetitions. If you still have plenty of gas left in your tank, head for 30 or 40.

Rest as long as you feel you need to. Don't restrict yourself to 60 seconds or, worse still, 30 seconds, just because someone somewhere said that that is the right amount of time between sets. Your individual response to exercise, and the degree of systemic fatigue you experience from it, are highly individualized. Your recovery ability from an all-out set of strongest-range standing presses could well be closer to 3 minutes—or more! So train at your own pace as dictated by your Power Factor and Power Index numbers.

Barbell Shrug

This exercise directly involves the trapezius muscles of your upper back as well as your entire shoulder structure, so the combined muscular effect will enable you to move some tremendous poundages. You will need to perform this movement in a Power Rack for total safety and confidence. It is strongly advisable to get yourself a pair of heavy-duty lifting hooks to be used during the performance of this exercise, as the tonnage you'll be hoisting in this movement will mount up very quickly.

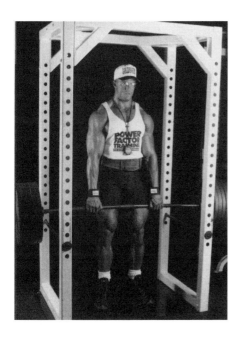
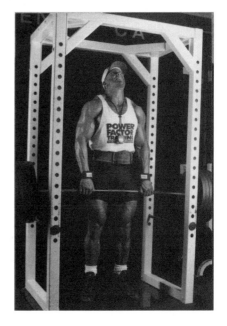

Barbell shrug—start position   *Barbell shrug—finish position*

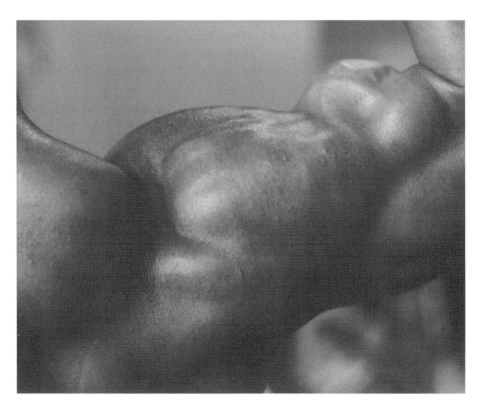

The barbell shrug directly involves the trapezius muscles of your upper back, as well as your entire shoulder structure.

1. To begin this movement, place the safety bars of the Power Rack in a position that allows the bar to rest two to four inches below your hands if you are standing up straight inside the Power Rack. Take an overhand grip on a barbell and, after establishing that your grip and footing is secure, stand erect inside the Power Rack, thereby pulling the weight up off the pins. Your hands should be slightly wider apart than your shoulders.

2. Once you're standing upright, begin to shrug your shoulders upward as quickly as possible with no pause at either the top or the bottom of the move-

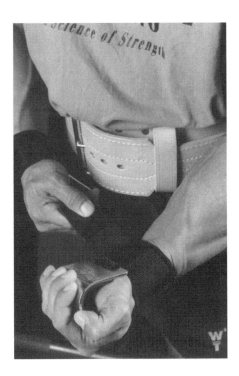

It is strongly advisable to get yourself a pair of heavy-duty lifting hooks to use during the performance of this exercise. The tonnage you'll be hoisting in this movement will mount up very quickly.

ment. Use a range of motion that is one-half, or slightly less, than your full range.

Again, get that nice, quick cadence going. Remember, the more work or reps you perform in a given set, the greater your muscle growth stimulation. Make the movement like a sprint with weights. Keep it going until you cannot draw the weight up even a fraction of an inch. Make sure to keep your arms straight at all times to ensure that your traps alone, not your biceps, are doing the work.

Close-Grip Bench Press

The close-grip bench press imparts tremendous overload on the triceps as well as pectorals and anterior deltoids, thereby stimulating phenomenal upper-body muscle growth.

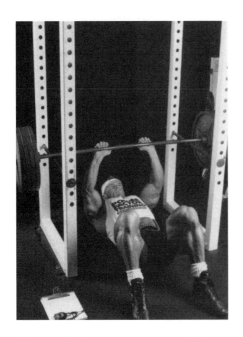

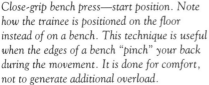

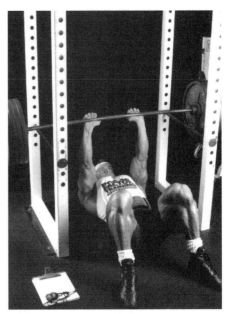

Close-grip bench press—start position. Note how the trainee is positioned on the floor instead of on a bench. This technique is useful when the edges of a bench "pinch" your back during the movement. It is done for comfort, not to generate additional overload.

Close-grip bench press—finish position

1. To start, place the safety bars of the Power Rack in a position that allows the bar to rest two to four inches below your full reach. When you are a newcomer to strongest-range training, you can place the bar a full six inches under your fully extended reach. Once you're comfortable handling the heavier poundages, decrease the distance of travel to two to three inches.

2. Take a narrow overhand grip in the middle of a barbell (with the outside of your palms just touching the inside of the knurling). Lying on your back on a flat bench inside the Power Rack, raise the barbell off the pins and extend your arms upward until they are completely locked out.

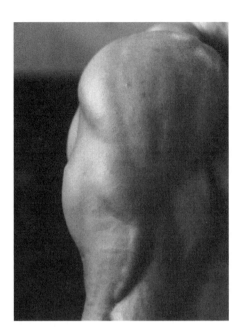

The close-grip bench press predominately stimulates the triceps muscles of your upper arm.

3. From this fully extended position, bend your elbows slightly, just lowering the barbell an inch or two downward, then push it back up to the starting position.

    Again, it's important to get a good cadence going with this exercise until you're at the upper limits your individual Power Factor will allow.

Preacher Curl
Partial-range barbell Preacher curls will provide tremendous overload to the biceps muscles of your upper arms primarily and your brachialis and forearm muscles secondarily.

1. To begin, take a shoulder-width underhanded grip on either a cambered or regular barbell. Anchor your elbows firmly onto the pad on the top of the Preacher bench and keep them there throughout

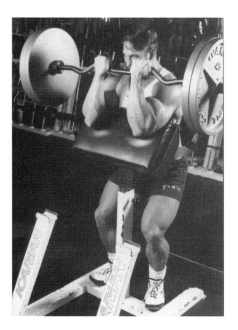
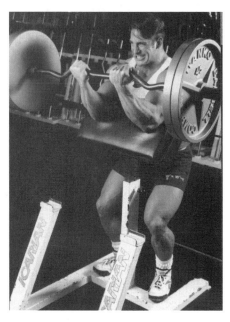

Preacher curl—start position   Preacher curl—finish position

the duration of the exercise. The bench itself should be at a ninety-degree angle to the floor (if possible) in order to ensure maximum resistance in the fully contracted position. Lean back slightly to generate even more power.

2. Either clean the barbell via "cheat curl" to your shoulders or, better yet, have a training partner or assistant help you lift the barbell up into the fully contracted position for you.

3. Lower the barbell slightly, about three inches, then immediately reverse the procedure and, pulling with biceps power alone, bring the barbell back up to the fully contracted position.

As with all these exercises, pyramid your weight for each set until you have performed the last set to failure with the heaviest weight.

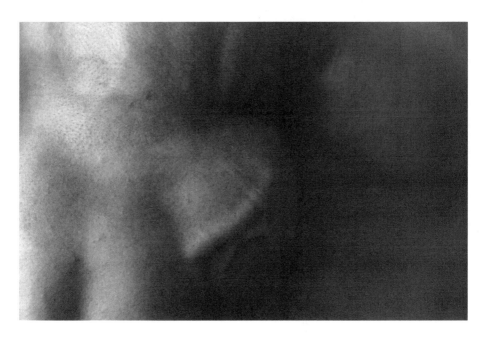

Preacher curls will provide tremendous overload to the biceps muscles of your upper arms.

Weighted Crunch

Crunches are the best abdominal-specific exercise. Your abs will get considerable use through their supporting role in the other exercises like standing barbell presses, but if you really want to specifically target them, this is the exercise.

1. To begin, lie on your back on the floor, with your hands behind your head and your feet on top of a bench. Take hold of the crunch strap, which should be attached to a low pulley.
2. Trying to keep your chin on your chest, slowly curl your trunk upward toward a sitting position. Make sure you hold onto the strap tightly so that your abdominals are contracting maximally against the resistance. You'll find that you can only curl up a third of the range you would if performing a normal

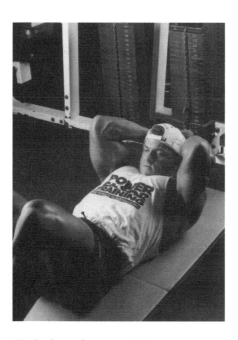

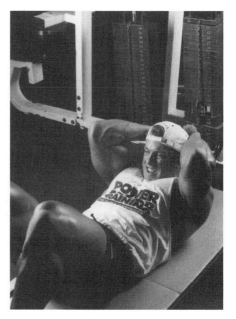

Weighted crunch—start position

Weighted crunch—finish position. Note that the weight stack has moved three to four inches.

sit-up. This is fine because that is all the range of motion that your abdominals require to be stimulated into maximum growth.

3. Once you have ascended to a fully contracted position, hold the position for a two count and then lower yourself slowly back to the starting position. Repeat for the required number of repetitions.

That's the end of Workout A. You will notice with Power Factor Training a sense of deep tissue fatigue, as opposed to a superficial pump. This fatigue indicates that your muscles and the nervous system that supplies them have been called upon to perform tasks that heretofore have never been attempted. You will also notice an increase in appetite and, when you go to bed, a deep and sound sleep pattern. When it comes time to repeat this

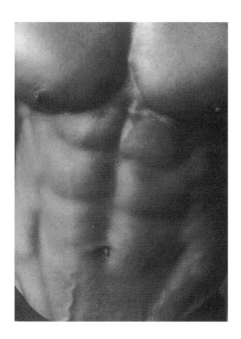

Weighted crunches are the best abdominal-specific exercise that we have measured. They deliver great results.

workout, you will, if you took enough time off between training sessions, be stronger. In fact, your strength—as measured by your Power Factor and Power Index—should be increasing dramatically with every workout.

WORKOUT B

When starting out, perform 2 sets of 20 repetitions for each of the following exercises. Once again, increase the resistance with each succeeding set.

Dead Lift

The dead lift is the greatest exercise you can perform for developing the muscles of your lower back, buttocks, and hamstrings. Always keep a slight bend in your knees when performing this exercise in order to insure that your lumbar muscles, rather than your vertebrae, bear the brunt of the exercise stress.

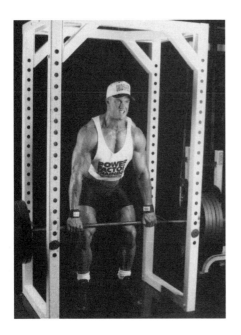

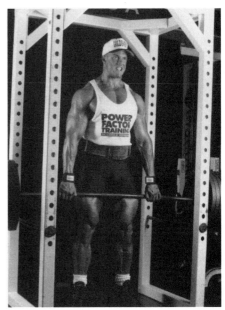

Dead lift—start position   *Dead lift—finish position*

1. Start by placing a barbell inside the Power Rack at
   a height just slightly above your knees. Stand inside
   the Power Rack and grasp the barbell with a grip of
   approximately shoulder width. Your feet should be
   under the bar.
2. Slowly pull the resistance upward, making sure to
   keep your arms straight, until you are fully erect
   and the barbell is resting on your upper thighs.
3. From this fully erect position, lower the barbell
   smoothly, bending at the waist approximately four
   to five inches—if you're a newcomer to strongest-
   range training—while keeping a slight bend in your
   knees throughout the movement.
4. Then raise the weight back up to the starting position, using only the power of your hamstrings,
   glutes, and lower back muscles. If you are already

accustomed to the demands and mechanics of strongest-range training, shorten the range of travel to about three inches.

Once the range has been shortened, you'll need even heavier weights to fully recruit the fibers of your spinal erectors, glutes, and even your deltoids. This is fine, as training in your strongest range will allow you to exercise in the safest possible range of motion while the extra-heavy weights employed will recruit even more muscle fibers. The more fibers you can recruit, the more growth stimulation you'll be imparting.

Bench Press

As most bodybuilders are aware, the bench press is a fundamental compound movement for the upper body. When

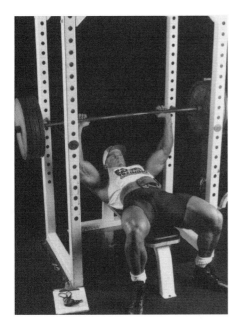 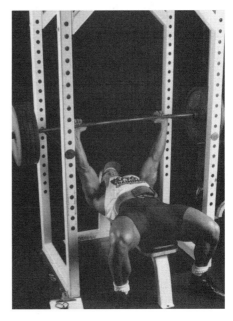

Bench press—start position   *Bench press—finish position*

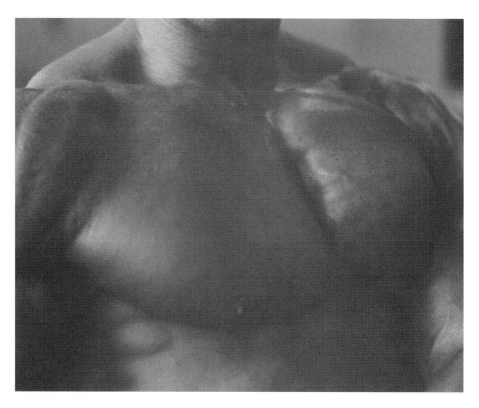

The bench press is a fundamental compound movement for the upper body that will build incredible power, mass, and strength into the chest.

performed exclusively through its strongest range of motion, it will build incredible power, mass, and strength into the pectorals, anterior deltoids, and triceps muscles.

1. Start by lying back on a flat bench inside a Power Rack. Set the pins in the rack to three to four inches below your full lockout reach. Place your feet flat on the floor for balance. Your grip should be medium width so that, as you lower the bar, your forearms are straight up and down (vertical).
2. Raise the barbell from the pins and lock it out directly above your chest. With the bar directly

above your chest, lower the bar until there's a slight bend in your elbows—not such a bend that the barbell touches the pins in the Power Rack, but enough that it comes close to touching.

3. Press the barbell upward until your arms are fully locked out again. Repeat for 4 sets of 10 to 30 repetitions, adding weight with each successive set.

Your rep cadence on this and all other exercises will be as quick as possible so as to get you your highest possible Power Factor and Power Index.

Lat Pulldown
The lat pulldown will widen your upper lats and put you well on your way to developing an incredible V shape. It also allows you to utilize more weight than your

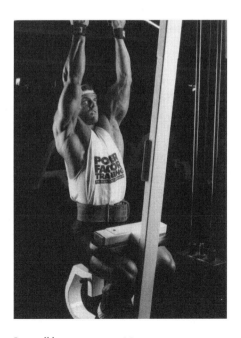
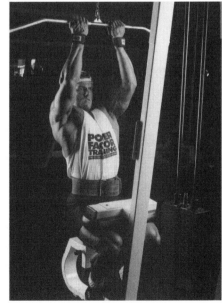

Lat pulldown—start position   *Lat pulldown—finish position*

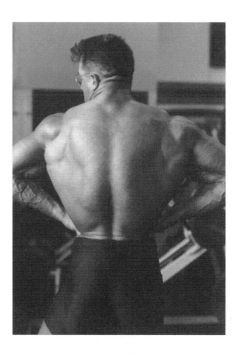

Pulldowns will widen your upper lats and put you well on your way to developing an incredible V shape.

bodyweight can provide. For overload purposes, this can prove to be a very desirable factor.

1. To begin, take a close, underhand grip on the bar. Sit on the seat with your knees hooked under the support. Your arms should be stretched fully above your head, and you should feel the pull in both your lats and shoulder blades.

2. Pull the bar just slightly down—about three to four inches of travel—then return it to the starting position. As you increase your weight, reduce your range of travel by just pulling on the bar and making it move two or three inches by the force of contracting your lats alone. Concentrate on making

the upper back do the work, and don't lean backward to involve the lower back.

3. Release the contraction and make a point of feeling the lats return to the fully stretched position.

Leg Press

The leg press involves extensive use of the quadriceps, hamstrings, and buttocks. Because of the tonnage your legs can support in this movement, it is one of the best exercises that can be used in Power Factor Training. Leg presses permit the use of weight that is much heavier than most people can safely squat.

1. To begin, sit down in a leg press machine with your back pressed comfortably against the angled pad and your buttocks on the seat bottom. Place your feet on the sled with your heels about shoulder width apart and your toes pointed either straight ahead or angled slightly outward.

2. Straighten your legs and release the stop bars of the machine (or keep them locked if you are long-legged). Grasp the handles beside the seat or the

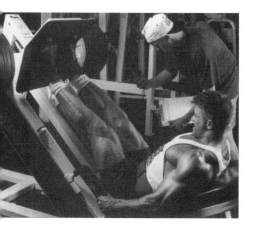
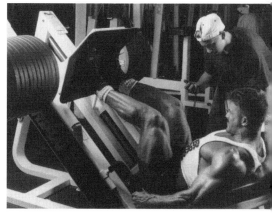

Leg press—start position   *Leg press—finish position*

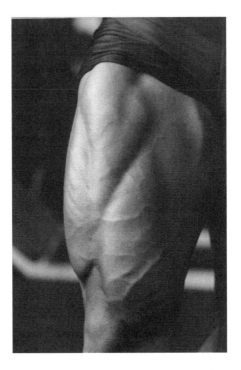

The leg press builds powerful quadriceps and hamstrings in your upper legs.

edge of the seat itself for better balance during the movement.

3. Once the weight has been pressed upward and your straightened legs are just short of a full lockout, lower the weight about two to three inches, then reverse the movement and press it back up to the starting position.

Never throw the weight upward or let it drop downward. Instead, perform each and every repetition under complete control over the limited range of motion. If you're just beginning, a range of four to six inches might feel more comfortable.

Toe Press on Leg Press Machine

The toe press is a great exercise for the gastrocnemius (calf) and associated muscles of the lower leg, as it allows you to pile on (in some instances) a ton of poundage!

1. To begin, sit in a leg press machine the same way you would if you were about to perform a standard set of leg presses. Place your feet on the platform, and slowly push with your legs until your knees are locked out and your legs are straight.
2. Once you have fully extended your legs, carefully slide your heels off the platform until only your toes and the balls of your feet remain in contact with it. Whenever possible, keep the machine's lock pins in place while performing this exercise as an added safety precaution in case your feet should slip off the platform.

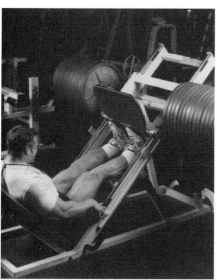 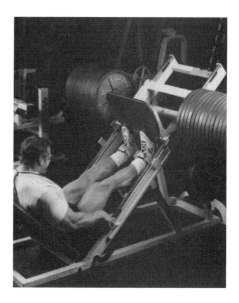

Toe press—start position   *Toe press—finish position*

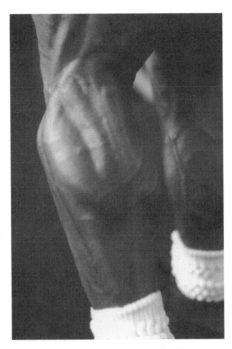

The toe press is a great exercise for the gastrocnemius (calf) and associated muscles of the lower leg. It allows you to pile on, in some instances, a ton of poundage.

3. Keeping your legs straight, allow the weight of the machine to force your toes back slightly toward your body, then contract your calves, completely extending your toes. The range here is limited to one or two inches of travel, whether you are a beginner or an advanced trainee.
4. Add weight each set, duplicating the cadence and repetition scheme used in the strongest-range leg presses just discussed.

Don't forget: Train by the numbers, and you'll make continual, uninterrupted progress until you've reached the outermost limits of your genetic potential. And if that means only one workout every two weeks, so what? If that's what it takes for you to record a strength and size increase, then that's what it takes, and there's no getting around it.

If you trained with sufficient progressive overload, you will be a stronger person when you return to the gym. Don't perform the identical workout next time, as it will be too low an intensity for your increased strength.

SUBSTITUTE EXERCISES

Over the years we have learned there are a number of exercises that some people have found to be maximally effective. Some, too, are forced to make substitutions because of limited equipment availability.

Partial squats are an excellent exercise in their own right. They do require more finesse than leg presses and

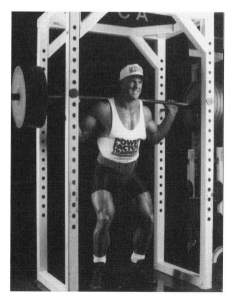

Partial squat—start position

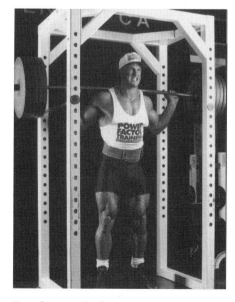

Partial squat—finish position

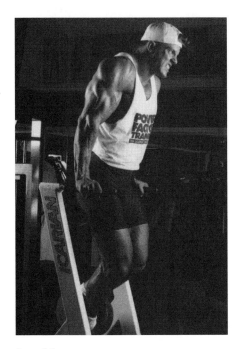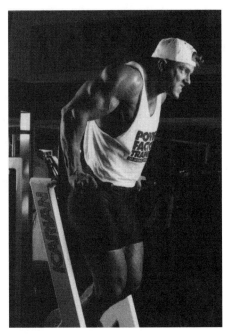

Partial dips—start position   *Partial dips—finish position*

are therefore more prone to cause injury. But if you have no leg press available, they are a good substitute.

For triceps many have found good results from performing weighted partial dips. The weighted aspect is important because it permits progressive overload, whereas standard dips do not. Cable pushdowns also are excellent, but they do not allow you to progress to weight above your bodyweight.

For the lats some people perform weighted partial chins or use a low pulley and a partial (two- to four-inch) rowing motion, using only the lats (not the biceps) to pull. Also, some people have resorted to one-armed lat pulldowns when their strength with both hands exceeded the available weight stack.

For the lower back we have discovered that some people who can't perform dead lifts prefer a low pulley

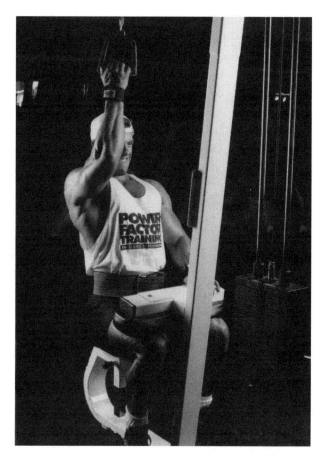

One-armed lat pulldowns can be used when your strength with both arms exceeds the weight of the entire stack. That's a common problem with Power Factor trainees!

row in which the arms are locked forward (not used) and the lower back muscles are used to lean back two to four inches.

In principle, you can make any substitution you like. The key is to use the best exercise (or at least the best available) to generate the highest overload for the targeted muscle or muscle group. Let your numbers be your guide.

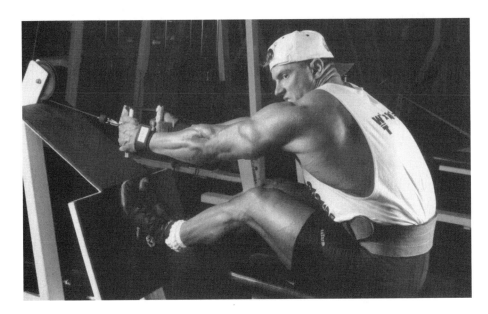

Low pulley lat—start position

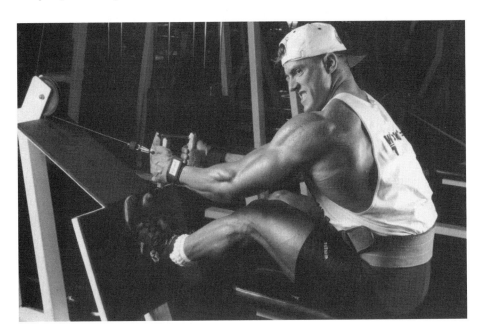

Low pulley lat—finish position

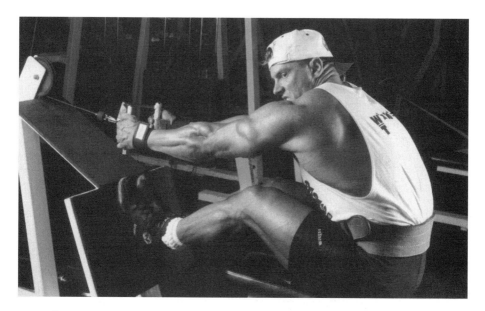

Low pulley back—start position

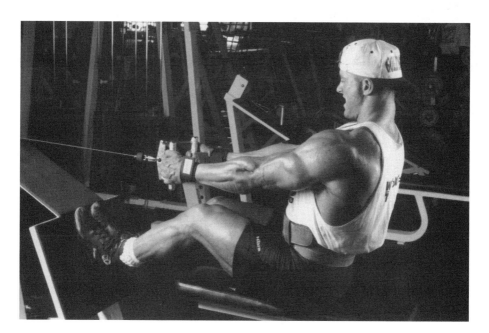

Low pulley back—finish position

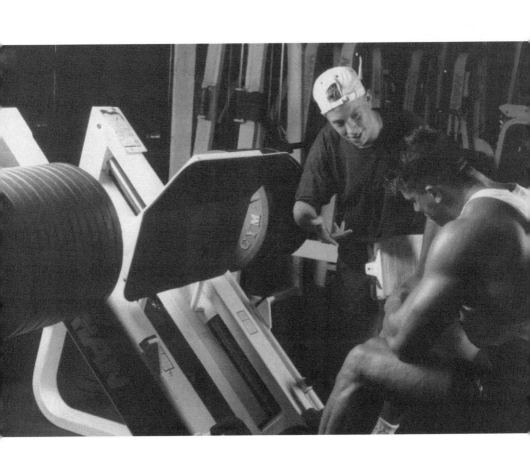

10

Recovery Ability: The Forgotten Factor

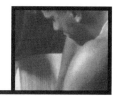

Exercise physiologists have found that strength increases occur only when the athlete's amount of training and recovery ability are in balance. Because this balance is both delicate and elusive, it can be established and sustained only if you understand the intricacies involved in the three-phase process of recuperation.

If you return to the gym too soon after a workout, you will not perform as well, and your numbers will reflect this.

THE GROWTH PROCESS

Phase 1 of systemic recovery takes place in the minutes and hours immediately after an intense workout. Some exercise physiologists have theorized that within as little as three seconds after a muscle has been worked to a point of momentary muscular failure, it can recover a substantial portion of the strength it lost as a result of the exercise. (It is during this immediate phase that most of the local energy reserves utilized in the actual training effort are replenished.) However, this does not mean that the muscle will recover its full capacity nor the deeper reserves of general adaptation energy in six seconds or even in as many minutes. When and only when this initial phase has been completed, the regeneration process can begin the additional repair, growth, and strengthening of the muscles themselves.

The second phase is chemical in nature, and it is rather time-consuming. Current research makes it clear that what had previously been considered a mandatory recovery period between workouts of forty-two to sixty hours may have missed the side of the barn by at least seven days. In some cases, up to six weeks may be required for Phase 2 to successfully run its course (depending, of course, on the type and amount of overload imposed on the system and individual recovery ability).

Phase 3, that of overcompensation or muscle growth, takes place only when the previous two phases have elapsed. Any additional training undertaken before Phases 1 and 2 are complete will be with a muscular system that has been denied full recuperation and growth. If this approach is repeated regularly, strength will decrease. This is why allowing for adequate recovery and growth is absolutely crucial to your continued progress.

THE TWO SIDES OF RECOVERY

Like all other physical characteristics of humans, recovery ability after exercise varies very widely among individuals. After identical workouts, one person may be able to return to the gym in forty-eight hours and see an increase in his Power Factor and Power Index, while another person may need a full week in order to recover sufficiently and show improvement.

When you use Power Factor Training, you will be able to see the extent to which you have recovered by virtue of your Power Factor and Power Index. If you return to the gym too soon after a workout, you will not perform as well, and your numbers will reflect this. When this happens, just add a day or two of recovery until your numbers show some improvement.

As alluded to earlier, this newfound ability led us to an entirely different perspective on recovery ability. During the development of Power Factor Training, each of us at one time had to take six weeks off from working out. When we finally returned to the gym, we were mentally prepared for a light workout. To our surprise, however, we discovered that, as the workout progressed, we not only had no sign of atrophy but our strength had taken a quantum leap upward. In fact, we both set new personal records in every lift we performed.

It is clear that recovery can be measured along a range of time that begins with the first day you can return to the gym and expect an improvement and ends with the last day you can return to the gym and expect an improvement. Power Factor Training will allow you to precisely determine your personal range of recovery. Depending on a variety of personal factors, your own range may be anywhere from two or three days to many weeks.

Consequently, if you are the sort of person who loves to train and wants to be in the gym as frequently as possible, you can work at the close end of your range of recovery scale by returning to the gym as soon as you are able. If, on the other hand, you have family or business commitments or an otherwise busy schedule, you can schedule your workouts further apart by working at the far end of your recovery range and working out as little as possible without losing ground as measured by your Power

Factor and Power Index. In either case, you'll make dramatic and consistent progress.

PROTRACTED RECOVERY PERIODS

The value of knowing your personal range of recovery ability is that you'll know, with mathematical precision, exactly when you honestly do have to train and when you don't. Somebody else's ability to train three days a week and make progress is irrelevant in your personal training considerations. He may have stumbled onto a margin of training that falls within his range of personal recovery ability and is (for the moment, at least) making progress. His problem will arise when he eventually ceases to make progress. He won't know if his lack of progress is due to having reached the upper limits of his genetic potential, having become "stale," or having trained with insufficient intensity to continue the growth process.

On the other hand, if you know how many days it takes you to recover from having lifted *x* pounds in a given workout, then it stands to reason that it will take even more days to recover once you've increased your Power Factor. No longer do you need to entertain guilty thoughts because you didn't train one day last week. The truth of the matter is that you would have been doing more harm than good to your strength and physique aspirations if you worked out even one day sooner than the first day that your recovery ability had replenished itself.

What we've learned about recovery ability is that the body has a general and very limited supply, almost like a small reservoir. Every time you lift a weight, you dip into this reservoir a certain percentage—a percentage that must ultimately be replaced before the growth process can occur. In fact, some exercise physiologists have theorized that while the average trainee has the potential to increase his starting level of strength some 300 percent within the first year of training, his ability to recover from such workouts increases by only 50 percent. The trainee's rate of overloading his system increases at a different rate than his ability to recover from the overload, thereby posing a fundamental challenge.

Think of it this way. Say that your body has the ability to recover from 100 units of exercise per day. When you start your training, your strength is minimal, and you may be capable of generating only 70 or 80 units of overload. No problem; your metabolic system can recover from that in one day. As you grow stronger, however, your muscles can generate 150 units of overload, which will take two days to recover from. By the time your recovery ability begins to improve, your muscular output might be up to 300 to 350 units of overload, and you must take multiple days off between workouts. This is a critical balance; the trainee who returns to the gym too soon will have a recovery deficit that has not been paid off in sufficient recovery units and will just dig himself a bigger hole from which to recuperate.

When you use Power Factor Training, you will be able to see the extent to which you have recovered by virtue of your Power Factor and Power Index numbers. If you return to the gym too soon after a workout, you will not perform as well, and your numbers will reflect this. When this happens, just add a day or two of recovery until your numbers show some improvement.

MENTZER'S RESEARCH

At about the time the authors encountered their first plateau on the Power Factor Training system, Mike Mentzer, former Mr. Universe, called to inform us of the results of some recent research he had conducted over a two-year period involving some 200 clients who had been training under his direct supervision:

> *I've noted with many of my clients that they're stronger after a two- to three-week layoff. I've noted this with all of my clients, some of whom were either forced to take a layoff or had to for a variety of other reasons. Almost all of them expressed an anxiety of, "Geez, I'm afraid I'm going to lose my size and strength if I take time off from training," but I've had these people take up to three weeks off, and with almost every single case, they've come back stronger. I even asked [Mr. Olympia] Dorian Yates whether or not he'd noted a similar phenomenon with regard to his own training experience, and he said, "You know, Mike, it's true."*
>
> *This is not just a minor point to be glossed over. I'm beginning to suspect this thing with frequency of training has a hell of a lot to do with a trainee's ulti-mate success. Maybe the solution would be to train each body part once every two weeks. Why not?*[1]

Why not indeed? As Mentzer has correctly pointed out in his articles in *Muscle & Fitness* and *Flex* magazines (as well as in his 1996 book *Heavy Duty II*), training progress should not be an unpredictable, haphazard, irreg-ular phenomenon. If you're training with sufficient over-load to stimulate growth and allowing (what for you is) adequate recovery time to take place, then you should be witnessing consistent improvement on a regular basis. Conversely, if you're training with inadequate overload and too frequently, you will short-circuit both the recov-ery and growth processes.

OVERTRAINING AND CELLULAR DAMAGE

The clinical evidence that we need to train less frequently is finally starting to trickle in from the medical community. In fact, research conducted by Michael Sherman back when he was a research associate at Ball State University in Indiana strongly indicates that rest and recovery goes way beyond simply allowing ourselves to feel better; it's also absolutely essential to the cells of our bodies. In the January 1985 issue of *American Health* magazine, Stephen Kiesling had this to say about Sherman's research:

> *When Sherman aimed an electron microscope at the leg-muscle cells of marathon runners, he saw "twisted cells, torn cells, and cells turned inside out." And that was the day-before-the-race damage from training. The day after the event, even more cells were battered.*
>
> *In a related experiment, Sherman found that even after a full week of rest, marathon runners had not regained pre-race strength and power. Returning to moderate running after the marathon delayed recovery. And some races may take months to recover from.*[2]

While this study was performed on marathon runners, who admittedly are the extreme example of high-volume training, it could just as easily have been applied to bodybuilders who train twice a day, six to seven days per week with high-volume and often ballistic training methods. According to Mentzer, bodybuilders may even be at greater risk, owing to the higher overloads with which they routinely train:

*You've got to be real careful whenever you're
training at peak overload levels. What I'm beginning to see much more clearly is just how demanding this stuff is. Arthur Jones said some years ago,
"For every slight increase in intensity, there has to
be a disproportionate decrease in volume," and he
wasn't joking.*

*High-intensity training places a demand on the
body of an order that is phenomenal. If you were to
draw a horizontal line from left to right across a
sheet of paper with that line representing zero effort
and then, off of that line, graph your daily effort
output such as getting up in the morning, brushing
your teeth, walking to your car, climbing some
steps to get to work, etc., the graph representing
that kind of effort output would barely leave the flat
line. It would be a little squiggly sine wave. Then
you go into the gym and perform a heavy set of partial bench presses. All of a sudden that little squiggly line would start to take off in a straight vertical
line—off the paper, out the door, down the street,
and around the block! Within the space separating
that peak of vertical ascent from the flat line is how
much more biochemical resources have been used
up. Do you see how dramatic a difference that is?[3]*

The conclusion to draw from Mike Mentzer's experience and Michael Sherman's research is simply that overtraining is a very real problem and that the actual process
of working out makes far greater systemic demands and
creates far more cellular damage than was previously
believed. Additionally, their work and ours has revealed
that it is far easier to overtrain than was previously
believed. Further, the recovery process, which always pre-
cedes the growth process, can take upwards of one full

week to complete (and perhaps much longer), and training before the bi-phasic process of recovery and growth has taken place will result in, at minimum, slower progress and, in the worst case, dangerous physical exhaustion.

STRESS AND ADAPTATION

The whole issue of recovery ability might be made more lucid if we look at it in terms of the body's capacity to cope with stress. Up to a certain point, for example, exposure to the sun will lead to the formation of a tan. While our reason for tanning is a purely cosmetic one, the actual process of acquiring a tan is a perfect example of how our bodies adapt to protect our tissues from the stressor of ultraviolet light.

The adaptive process, whether in response to ultraviolet light or progressive-overload weight training, is essentially defensive. And the degree to which the process of adaptation is stimulated is directly proportional to the strength of the stressor. To follow through on our suntanning example, if you decide to lie out in the sun in the middle of January, you can remain outside all day long and show little or nothing in the way of a tan for your efforts. The reason is that the sun is not directly overhead at this time of year and, correspondingly, its rays are not as intense. The sun's rays must be of a certain strength in order to elicit an adaptive response from our bodies (in this case, the marshaling of the body's store of melanin, or skin pigment).

Conversely, when you decide to lie out in the hot sun in the middle of July, you don't have to wait hours, days, or weeks to see results (that is, to stimulate an adaptive response). Rather, it's an immediate occurrence that is directly proportionate to the intensity or strength of the stressor (the sun that is now directly overhead). Your skin gets red and slightly inflamed, and the tanning process is almost instantaneous.

While it's beyond our immediate power to control the strength of the sun's rays, which depend upon the seasons, weight training happens to be a form of bodily stress over which we have direct control. The level of weight training overload depends solely upon our ability and willingness to generate the necessary effort required to overload our muscles.

Just as the sun is a form of stress to the skin, Power Factor Training is a form of stress to the muscles and the overall physical system. Heavy-overload exercise, when not performed to excess, will stimulate a compensatory buildup in the form of added muscle tissue, which aids the body in coping more successfully with similar stressors in the future. However, taken to extremes—as in the case of excessive exposure to the strong summer rays of the sun, which causes the skin to blister and decompensate, or break down—bodybuilders who insist on training six to seven days a week will witness a similar decompensatory effect. The resulting drain on the body's regulatory subsystems will actually prevent the buildup of muscle. In fact, all of the energy reserves will have to be utilized in an attempt to overcome the energy debt caused by overexposure to training.

SYMPTOMS OF OVERTRAINING

A trainee who has entered an overtrained state has many telltale symptoms of this condition. One of these is an almost constant sense of fatigue combined with a deep lack of energy and ambition. According to Dr. Gabe Mirkin in *The Sports Medicine Book*, chronic fatigue accompanied by frequent colds and injuries is a sure sign that you've overdone it. Mirkin lists these other signs as further indicators of overtraining:

- Persistent soreness and stiffness in the muscles, joints, or tendons
- Heavy-leggedness
- Loss of interest in training
- Nervousness
- Depression—"I don't care" attitude
- Inability to relax
- Decrease in academic work or performance
- Sleep problems
- Headache
- Loss of appetite
- Fatigue and sluggishness
- Loss of weight
- Swelling of the lymph nodes in the neck, groin, and armpit
- Constipation or diarrhea
- In women, the absence of menstruation

One of the popular methods used to detect overtraining is to monitor the morning pulse rate. Upon arising, the athlete takes his pulse for sixty seconds. If it is seven beats a minute faster than usual, a layoff or reduction in training is indicated. Perhaps the most blatant symptom of overtraining is a very strong disinclination to train at all. Your body is signaling your brain that it hasn't fully recovered from the cumulative systemic toll of previous training sessions. Any person who falls into the habit of training five and six days a week over prolonged periods of time will inevitably become overtrained, regardless of how powerful or well built that individual may be.

Eventually, as you become stronger and are able to utilize even greater overload in your training sessions, you will find that training even three days per week will prove to be too much. At this point, we recommend that you drop your weekly workouts to two, working half of the body in each one, so that each body part gets trained once per week. As you again progress, you may need to decrease your training frequency to one workout per week and, later still, to one workout every two weeks.

It's true that many bodybuilders who have been training for years never experience a state of overtraining and dismiss the notion as something that can't happen to them. However, in nine cases out of ten, the reason why they don't become overtrained is simply that they lack the drive to train with the requisite overload and effort to ever reach a condition of staleness. Plateaus are things that have to be progressed to—and from which all progress halts. To make progress, one must be willing to train with very high intensity. And that is something these people—who don't make any perceptible progress from year to year, let alone from workout to workout—will never achieve.

HOW TO COMBAT OVERTRAINING

As we now know what overtraining is, the question then becomes, How do you get rid of the overtraining symptoms once you've acquired them? The truth of the matter is that the problem is an individual one. Each trainee is obliged to consider his own case on its own merits. However, some general or basic rules apply to all human beings.

First off, there are varying degrees of overtraining. For example, a bodybuilder can train for a month or two and make steady gains in both power and physique. Then all at once he'll cease progressing and, even though he eats plenty of nourishing foods, his bodyweight will not increase. He may have been driving himself to the limit in his training, striving to add a single repetition or a couple of pounds, yet fail continually to gain them.

There is only one thing to do in a case like this, and fortunately it works. Simply take a short layoff from training. The lifter or bodybuilder not only needs freedom from his heavy-overload routine, he also needs freedom from all of the mental stress that goes along with training: psyching for lifts, resolving to shatter personal bests, that sort of thing. In short, the trainee would do well to forget about training entirely and focus instead on attempting to cultivate a stress-free mental environment, rest as much as possible, get as much sleep as he can (at least eight hours a night), and also try to get out into the fresh air as much as possible.

Stress-free pastimes such as movies or reading books, listening to music, and companionship can help hasten the recovery from overtraining almost as much as the rest itself. Diet at this time should be high in proteins and carbohydrates. Fresh fruits, salads, vegetables, and certain dried fruits such as seedless raisins will also prove beneficial in this respect. A multivitamin/mineral supplement with extra vitamins B (the so-called stress vitamin), C, and E can help as well.

Most sensible weight trainers take a layoff as soon as they observe a stale period coming on. As a result, they're able to stave it off before it hits and prevent any further serious symptoms from developing. In many cases, three or four days of rest from training will work wonders, and the trainee is soon ready to start back in again.

Instead of resting, however, some trainees try to train through their plateaus. They must remember that muscular soreness is not to be confused with overtraining. You can work soreness out of a muscle with a hard training session, but you can't get rid of overtraining by engaging in more work. In fact, just the reverse is true, and the condition of overtraining becomes exacerbated by the trainee's refusal to decrease his training. In severe cases, the trainee will have to lay off for as long as three to six months simply to recover from the exhaustive systemic affects that have accumulated.

Fortunately, these cases are rare. However, when they do occur, a long rest from weight training is an absolute must. Not only is the trainee's body in a state of chronic fatigue, but his nervous system and adaptation energy are in corresponding states of exhaustion and depletion. Continuing to force oneself to train for lengthy periods of time when a period of rest is needed will not only cause undue frustration and worry. If carried to extremes, it will result in a catabolic condition owing to both the over-work and accumulated stress. There is no reason to reach this state when using Power Factor Training, as steady declines in your Power Factor and Power Index will immediately indicate that you are training too frequently.

Other factors should be considered in overtraining. It would certainly behoove the trainee to remember these important physiological points:

- The greater the overload/intensity, the more rapid the approach of fatigue.
- Depending on the force output or work performed, if a sufficient rest interval is allowed between muscle contractions (that is, rest between sets), no great fatigue is apparent.
- Excessive outside stressors (those not induced by the workout) can hasten muscular fatigue, and vice versa.
- Marked fatigue in one group of muscles will diminish the capacity for work in other groups.
- Fatigue is reduced faster by rest, wholesome food, correct schedules of exercise, sufficient sleep, and proper stress management.

Take comfort in the fact that layoffs are temporary and the time will soon come when you can resume weight training. You should always have enthusiasm for lifting in order to succeed, since enthusiasm is a large part of the trainee's success. But it should be tempered somewhat, as unbridled enthusiasm can quickly lead to excessive training.

THE ABSOLUTE NECESSITY OF A TRAINING LOGBOOK

As there are so many factors to consider and so many variables encountered over the course of a training career, it's exceedingly difficult to remember all of the knowledge you have gathered from experience. It's doubtful that there exists any arena of human endeavor where a person discovers the most direct route to his destination right at the outset. Most learning and ultimate achievement are reached through a process of trial and error. By making a trial and missing the mark and then noting the error, you are then in a position to make the necessary adjustments. In so doing, you move closer to your goal.

For this reason, the proper application of Power Factor Training requires that you keep track of your workouts by recording frequency of exercise, exercises used, sets, reps, poundages, and times. This gives you an indicator of your progress and enables you to plan your next workout. According to Mike Mentzer, who kept a training logbook throughout his entire competitive career, "Becoming a massively developed bodybuilder takes time, a number of years in most cases. I do believe, however, that the amount of time it would take any person to develop to his fullest potential could be reduced

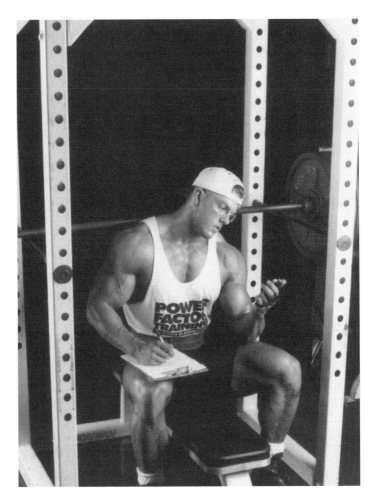

For the proper application of Power Factor Training, it is crucial to keep track of your workouts in your log.

dramatically if he were to keep a training journal from the day he began training."

If you view your training as a journey whose destination is the fulfillment of your physical potential, a training journal will serve as a sort of physiological road map. Keeping a proper record of every proper turn as well as every mistake made along the way can help you avoid the pitfalls that will slow down your progress. A training log-book serves as a historical record of your workouts, the recovery period that yielded the best progress between your workouts, and the timing of reductions in training volume and frequency. It should also include your daily caloric intake and the types of foods consumed. By recording your daily food consumption, you can calculate your nutritional requirements for future weight gain and loss, as well as observe the effects of different diets on peak performance output.

Charting your progress can yield invaluable training data. Eventually, you'll have enough information in your training logbook to make precise determinations of everything from overload volume to frequency of train-ing for optimal results.

NOTES

1. Mike Mentzer, in a conversation with John Little, November 1992.
2. Stephen Kiesling, *American Health* (January 1985).
3. Mike Mentzer, in a conversation with John Little.

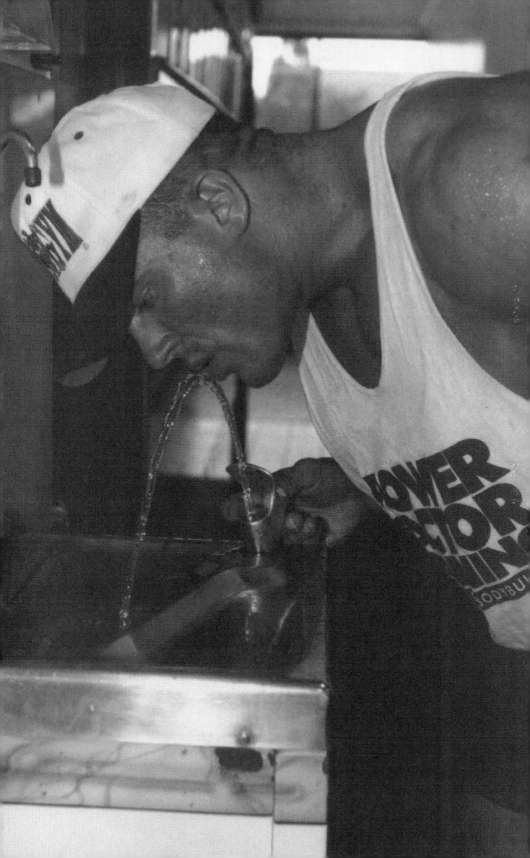

11

A Nutrition Seminar

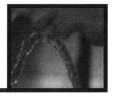

Although there is no magic number of muscular pounds you will gain by following the Power Factor Training method, it is a safe bet that the minimum amount of pure muscle that an average male could expect to gain after one year of such training would be 10 pounds. Although the material presented in this chapter is geared primarily toward gaining lean body mass, those who desire to lose weight or firm up will find the material contained herein of use as well.

Eat, drink, and get huge—with Power Factor Training.

We mention the figure of 10 pounds knowing full well that some readers have the capacity to gain three to four times this amount over a twelve-month period and could quite possibly gain 10 pounds of lean muscle mass in as little as three workouts. Nevertheless, for the sake of illustration, let's assume that you are a reasonably advanced trainee and have struggled for years trying to increase your muscle mass stores, yet you still weigh the same, month after month, year after year in spite of your efforts.

GAINING 10 POUNDS OF MUSCLE

Some exercise physiologists and experienced body-builders believe that gaining even 10 pounds of muscle a year would be a considerable achievement. Let it be understood right off the top that we're not referring here to simply gaining 10 pounds of bodyweight—that's a relatively simple procedure—but rather 10 pounds of pure muscle. On the surface, such an amount doesn't really sound like much to gain over a twelve-month period. But looked at over the long term—say, five years, which is how you have to look at a training career (as nobody ever became Mr. Olympia in one year)—gaining at that rate in five years you would gain 50 pounds of muscle, which is enough to transform the average adult male weighing 165 pounds into a 215-pound Mr. Olympia competitor. In fact, many Mr. Olympia competitors actually weigh much less than 215 pounds, and these men are, whether they choose to admit to it or not, the thoroughbreds (genetically speaking) of our species. Therefore, the aforementioned exercise physiologists and bodybuilders have concluded that the acquisition of 10 pounds a year through training is almost beyond the reach of most of us lesser mortals.

But let's assume that we are all going to train hard enough to gain 10 pounds of muscle this year. Granted, we don't always think in terms of a year or in blocks of five years. We think about daily progress, daily workouts, and so forth. And if you think 10 pounds of muscle growth in one year is slow, it's unbelievable how slow such growth computes to on a daily level!

If you divide 10 pounds of muscle by the number of days it took to gain it (that is, 365), you'll see that the daily weight gain comes out to 0.027 pound of muscle. This is the same as 12 grams, or less than half an ounce. That's not even enough to register on a bodyweight scale!

Think for a moment just how minuscule 12 grams of muscle gain per day is—and that's assuming you're gaining
10 pounds of muscle per year. It's ridiculously slow. And
yet, when we don't seem to be gaining fast enough, the
typical reaction is to increase our training time, increase
our intake of supplements, and so forth. However, these
things don't hasten the muscle growth process.

THE ROLE OF NUTRITION

Obviously, gaining 10 pounds of muscle (or more) is
going to require some nutrition. At the very least, it's
going to require enough nutrition to maintain health
through what is referred to as a well-balanced diet.
However, if you want to make sure that the weight you
gain is all muscle, the question becomes, How much food
will you have to eat to gain these 10 pounds of pure muscle without adding any fat?

To answer this, you must first be aware that one
pound of muscle tissue contains 600 calories. This is true
of all human beings whether I'm talking about you or
Arnold Schwarzenegger. If you were to surgically cut
away a pound of muscle tissue and place it in a device
known as a calorimeter, it would give off 600 calories of
heat. It follows logically from this that, if you want to
gain 10 pounds, you would have to consume 600×10—
or 6,000—calories a year over and above your maintenance need of calories. That's 6,000 extra calories a *year*,
not 6,000 extra calories a day.

Being what they are, bodybuilders don't tend to think
in terms of a year, as there exists a pervasive attitude that
things have to happen in terms of days. They want to
know how many calories extra we need on a daily basis.
To obtain this answer, divide those 6,000 calories by 365
(the number of days in a year). You come out with the

answer that to grow 10 pounds of muscle a year, you need approximately 16 extra calories a day over and above your maintenance need of calories.

You can get those 16 extra calories a day by taking two bites out of an apple. Yet how many bodybuilders do you know who force-feed themselves hundreds or even thousands of extra calories a day with the mistaken notion that in so doing, they're hastening the muscle growth process? The logic is almost too simplistic. If you eat more, you're going to grow faster, that's true. But what you'll be growing is fat. To grow 10 pounds of muscle, you can't eat 16 extra calories a day. The process of eating itself actually contributes nothing to the muscle growth process.

THE FIRST REQUISITE FOR MUSCLE GROWTH

Nutrition plays a role only after you've met the first requisite for muscle growth: you've got to stimulate your muscles to grow through your training. You have to provide adequate nutrition to maintain your existing physical mass, and then you've got to provide that tiny bit of extra nutrition to allow for that tiny bit of extra growth that might take place on a daily basis. And we say "might take place," because it will all depend on how successful your efforts were in the gym. Again, keep in mind how minuscule growth is on a daily basis to gain 10 pounds of muscle a year.

GETTING ENOUGH CALORIES FOR GROWTH TO TAKE PLACE

For practical purposes, the majority of trainees already eat more than they need to grow 10 pounds of muscle a year anyway. That's why so few of us have ultra-low bodyfat

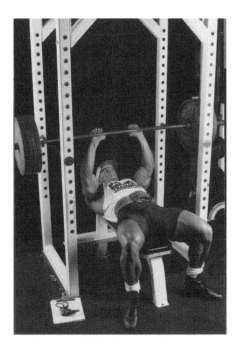

Never, never forget that the first requisite for muscle growth is to trigger the growth response through training.

(what we call being "ripped"). Most of us are actually eating too many calories as it is.

If you're not growing muscular mass now and you're eating sufficiently, what's the reason you're not growing? Answer: You're not stimulating growth in your training sessions. In short, you're not training with sufficient progressive muscular overload. Incidentally, very rarely is the answer to a muscular growth problem nutritional, particularly in North America, because almost everybody eats more than adequately.

We're not suggesting that you count your calories this exactly every day to make sure that you grow just muscular mass. What we're trying to point out by doing this arithmetic is that you don't have to force-feed yourself hundreds or even thousands of extra calories a day or hundreds of extra grams of protein. The notion that doing so will hasten the muscle growth process is simply mistaken.

DETERMINING YOUR MAINTENANCE NEED FOR CALORIES

Remember to allow for 10 pounds of muscle growth to manifest itself over the course of a year, you have to consume an additional 6,000 calories over and above your maintenance need of calories (given, of course, that you stimulated that growth in the first place). Also, there is a certain metabolic cost in the growth process, which may bump that extra caloric intake to 17 or 18 calories a day. (This is oversimplified, but it does give you some idea of just how slow the muscle growth process can be and how little additional supplementation or nutrition you really need to allow muscular growth to manifest.)

These calories are in addition to the calories you require every day to maintain your present bodyweight. At that specific amout of calories, referred to as your maintenance need, you don't gain weight and you don't lose weight. In sum, to grow an additional 10 pounds of muscle a year, you have to tack on 16 calories above your maintenance need on a daily basis. This simple procedure is, in essence, the nutritional "secret" to gaining muscular weight.

One way to discover your daily caloric needs is to multiply your present bodyweight by 10 and add to that either 10 percent, 15 percent, or 20 percent of that figure, depending on whether you are sedentary, moderately active, or very active. This is a fairly accurate rule of thumb to determine one's maintenance need of calories. But perhaps a more accurate way is to write down every single thing you eat, from the milk and sugar you put in your coffee to the dressing you put on your salads, over a random five-day period. It's important (for obvious reasons) that you don't change your diet during this period; you want to find out what your daily maintenance need of calories is. After each day, sit down with a calorie-counting book and calculate your total number of calories for that day. At the end of this five-day period, take your five daily totals, add them up, and divide this number by 5. The result will be your average daily maintenance need of calories, assuming you are not gaining or losing weight.

Try an example. Monday you consume 2,500 calories. On Tuesday you consume 2,700 calories. Wednesday is the middle of the week and you're getting tired and frustrated from your job, so you pig out and have 4,500 calories. On Thursday you feel guilty and decide to atone for your dietary aberrations, so you have only 1,500 calories.

On Friday you're back to normal, and you consume a more typical 2,500 calories. Add these five numbers (2,500 + 2,700 + 4,500 + 1,500 + 2,500 = 13,700 calories), then divide your total by the number of days involved (5). Your resulting average daily calorie intake is 2,740 calories per day. If over this five-day period you haven't gained or lost weight, it's your daily maintenance need of calories—the precise amount of calories you need to maintain your present bodyweight. If you want to gain 10 pounds of muscle a year, tack on 16 calories, and you would consume a grand total of 2,756 calories per day.

This procedure, incidentally, takes into account your individual basal metabolic rate (BMR) and your voluntary physical activity output. In other words, it doesn't matter how fast or slow your metabolism is; this method takes it into account. Your BMR is unique to you (that is, it's different for everybody), and it's factored into this method of determining your daily need of calories.

HOW MUCH PROTEIN YOU REALLY NEED

A lot of bodybuilders seem preoccupied with protein and how much extra protein is required to build muscle. Well, if we look again at our hypothetical example of growing 10 pounds of muscle a year, we see that it requires roughly 16 calories a day over and above our maintenance need of calories. As cited before, muscle tissue consists of approximately 25 percent protein. (It's actually 22 percent, but 25 percent is easier to remember and close enough.) Therefore, out of those 16 calories, about 4 (25 percent) should be protein calories. It just so happens that 1 gram of protein contains 4 calories, so to grow 10 pounds of muscle a year, you need to consume 1 gram of protein beyond your maintenance need of protein every day.

Some faddists honestly believe that if they don't have their hourly protein drink, their strength will decrease 50 pounds—and then it does, because they believe it. This power of suggestion is called the placebo effect. And contrary to what some believe, there are not some proteins that are more "anabolic." All proteins are broken down into the same essential elements—amino acids, glucose, fatty acids, etc. To be used by the human body, they're all broken down into exactly the same thing.

Also, contrary to much of what you've probably read, most of us already get more than enough protein from our diets. In fact, you'd have to look both long and hard to find trainees who are actually deficient in this macronutrient. Throughout North America and Europe, most people inadvertently ingest more protein than they need (except perhaps when the body's requirements rise under conditions, such as pregnancy, when bodyweight is elevated). There also exists evidence that consuming large quantities of protein may damage the kidneys and liver.

The metabolism and excretion of these nonstorable protein loads imposes major stress and can cause excessive growth of these vital organs.

You must understand that protein is not utilized to fuel your workouts. Bodybuilding workouts are fueled by glucose derived from carbohydrates. Cells and tissue, particularly muscle, are based on proteins, which are also an energy source. Barring a starvation diet, however, these proteins are spared for their primary purpose of tissue growth and repair. Individual protein requirements therefore depend solely upon individual bodyweight. Because protein is not normally a fuel source, your daily need for this macronutrient is not contingent upon how active you are in the gym.

McMaster University, one of Canada's leading exercise and nutrition science centers, recently released studies indicating that bodybuilders, who often consume up to three or four times the recommended daily intake of protein, actually need only 10 percent extra protein per day. In fact, according to the studies, joggers who log more than 100 kilometers (60 miles) a week need more protein than bodybuilders.

The researchers at McMaster University calculated daily protein requirements by monitoring intake and output of protein in the subjects' sweat, urine, and feces (and you thought a physiologist's work was all glamour and lecture circuits!). The recommended average daily intake for adults is 0.7 gram of protein per kilogram of bodyweight. For a 154-pound bodybuilder, this translates to about 49 grams of protein a day—the equivalent of sixteen ounces of milk, three ounces of chicken, five slices of bread, or four cups of spaghetti.

We can hear the cries of protest already: "But this figure of 0.7 is based on what the average individual requires, and bodybuilders work much harder than the average individual." Fine. So let's boost that percentage by 28.5 percent to 0.9 gram of protein per kilogram of bodyweight. (Remember that bodybuilders may be more active than the average man, but not that much more active, and the requirements depend on bodyweight, not activity level.) That same 154-pound bodybuilder now needs 63 grams of protein a day—only 14 more grams!

To determine your specific protein requirements, use the following method:

1. Divide your weight in pounds by 2.2 and round off the result to the nearest whole number. This is your approximate weight in kilograms.
2. Multiply this number by 0.9, our larger estimate of your protein need per kilogram.
3. The number that results is your specific daily protein requirement in grams.

Each time your bodyweight increases or decreases, you must recalculate your protein requirements. Failure to do so could upset your bodybuilding progress, as protein consumed in excess of the body's needs is either excreted (which represents a waste of money) or, worse, stored as fat (which represents, well, fat).

SUGAR: THE FUEL OF POWER FACTOR TRAINING

Power Factor Training, or any other form of weight training for that matter, doesn't burn all that many calories. And the calories that it does burn are sugar calories. It doesn't matter how you train, whether it's Power Factor Training or any other system. Any kind of weight training is considered a high-intensity activity, and all high-intensity activities depend entirely upon glucose as fuel.

So if you're trying to lose weight or lose fat to get cut up, weight training is the worst way to do it. Weight training uses 90 percent glucose for fuel, whereas aerobic activity will use up to 80 or 90 percent fat as fuel. If you're looking to get cut up, use Power Factor Training to either build or maintain your muscle mass, then spend the rest of your time doing aerobic activities to burn fat. This is not an opinion; it's a fact that can be backed up by any exercise physiologist or medical doctor.

THE BEST DIET TO FOLLOW
IN ORDER TO BUILD MASS

Simply eat a well-balanced diet. The most important aspect of eating a well-balanced diet is that it maintain health. This is something we all learned in eighth-grade health class. It also happens to be something we often forget. The first requisite in building a strong, healthy body is maintaining health—and the best way to maintain health is to eat a well-balanced diet.

A well-balanced diet comprises 60 percent carbohydrates, 25 percent protein, and 15 percent fats. If your daily maintenance need of calories is 3,000, out of those 3,000 calories, 60 percent should be carbohydrates, 25 percent protein, and 15 percent fats. This is how nutritional scientists and physical educators define a well-balanced diet. You will find quacks and faddists who say you should eat the majority of your calories from protein. In most instances those people also sell protein; they have a vested interest in distorting nutritional reality.

THE IMPORTANCE OF CARBOHYDRATES

Carbohydrates, next to water, are by far the most important nutritional element anybody, not just bodybuilders, could consume. The most important reason is that our nervous systems, our brains, our spinal cords, and our peripheral nerves derive 99.9 percent of their nutrition from the one thing that we've been taught is the worst thing we can eat: sugar. In fact, your brain derives 99 percent of its nutrition from sugar. Carbohydrates are the most important thing you can eat because they are the body's source of glucose, the sugar that is its basic fuel.

Anyone who goes on a low-carbohydrate diet notices a pronounced lack of energy almost immediately. They feel weak, tense, and edgy; they suffer impairment of concentration and short-term memory. They start dreaming about chocolate instead of sex. What are these signals? They're your nervous system sending out for the one thing it needs most: sugar!

If you've ever been around a bodybuilder who's been on a low-carb diet for six weeks or so, you'll see that it also impairs personality. Your personality's a product of your nervous system. If your nervous system is not getting the fuel it needs from carbohydrates, your personality is going to become altered. I've seen bodybuilders do weird things, and I've often wondered if this isn't the result of being on a low-carbohydrate diet for too long. Anybody who's been around bodybuilding for a long time, behind the scenes, knows that a lot of bodybuilders can seem crazy. They do strange things, and I think it's because of the one-time voguish low-carbohydrate diet. It affects the thinking process and personality. Low blood sugar will definitely cause an erratic personality; it's in all of the medical journals.

SIMPLE AND COMPLEX CARBOHYDRATES

By the time carbohydrates get into your bloodstream, they have to be in the form of glucose. Therefore, simple and complex carbohydrates give your body the same form of fuel. It makes no difference at all whether it's from a candy bar, an apple, a baked potato—the carbohydrate has to be in the form of glucose for your brain to use it.

However, it's not good to eat too many refined foods or simple sugars because they get into your bloodstream too fast and cause all kinds of problems. It's preferable to get your carbohydrates from as many natural sources as possible. The reason nutritional experts advocate that you try to get your carbohydrates from whole grains, fruits, and vegetables is that those foods lend themselves to a well-balanced diet. They contain vitamins and minerals and other important nutrients, along with fiber. But, if you have a hankering for an occasional candy bar, don't think the world's going to stop revolving.

HOW TO KNOW IF YOUR
DIET IS WELL BALANCED

If there's one issue in bodybuilding that's been confused, it's that of nutrition. Nutrition is really so simple; all you have to do is eat a well-balanced diet, which is really nothing more than consuming products from what used to be called the four basic food groups:

1. Fruits and vegetables
2. Cereals and grains
3. Dairy products
4. Meat, fish, and poultry

For a well-balanced diet, you should consume two to five portions from the first category, six to eleven portions from the second category, and only two to three portions from the final two categories. This may seem oversimplistic, but it's the truth of the matter. Even simpler, if you eat a little bit of everything but not too much of anything, you'll be getting a well-balanced diet. The matter of diet is really very simple.

Complicating the matter and confusing it are some of the crazy articles you read in some of the muscle magazines. These are designed solely to sell you more products by confusing you and muddying the issue. By adding to the confusion, they're able to divest you of your hard-earned dollars much more easily.

THE ROLE OF SUPPLEMENTS

When confronted with the nutritional basics, bodybuilders invariably wonder where supplements fit in. Well, if you're eating a well-balanced diet, then theoretically you don't need supplements because a well-balanced diet is just that: well balanced. By definition, you're getting everything you need—all the vitamins, minerals, carbohydrates, proteins, fats, and water you need to maintain health. However, it's often not possible to get a well-balanced diet due to time pressures, family pressures, job pressures, etc. We have to skip meals from time to time. If you suspect that you're not getting a well-balanced diet, then by all means include an all-around vitamin/mineral tablet or protein supplement.

However, there exists no need whatsoever to spend hundreds of dollars a month on useless vitamins and minerals that you're just going to pass through your system anyway. And you can see it, for example, if you take too much vitamin B; it will turn your urine bright yellow. Take supplements only when you think you may not be getting a well-balanced diet, such as before a contest while you're on a low-calorie diet. Once your calorie intake reaches a certain low level, you can't get a well-balanced diet. Some nutritional scientists say that once you go below 1,500 calories, it's impossible to get all the vitamins, proteins, minerals, and so forth that you need to maintain proper health and, of course, build a big, muscular physique.

Obviously, entire books can and have been written on nutritional supplements for bodybuilding. Often these books are written and/or published by someone selling nutritional supplements. Unfortunately, this is an area where products that might have some benefit to certain bodybuilders are advertised and sold right alongside purely fraudulent garbage. Sorting out the former from the latter can be a full-time job. Our best advice is to ignore all advertising claims, including testimonials, and instead consult a physician or registered dietitian.

THE MOST EFFICIENT FUEL
FOR BODYBUILDING

Carbohydrates are the most efficient fuel for Power Factor Training or any kind of anaerobic training. Anaerobic activity, which is what weight training is, demands sugar as fuel. Weight training does *not* burn fat as fuel (which is why it's the worst way to get defined muscularity). It's a simple medical fact that is not even open to debate. Weight training burns sugar, and if you're not getting sugar from fruits, vegetables, cereals, or grains, where is your muscle going to get sugar in order to continue contracting? If you're not getting dietary carbohydrates and you require sugar for high-intensity contractions, where is your body going to get sugar to continue contracting?

Answer: From your own muscle tissue! Your muscle tissue contains an amino acid called alanine, which will be broken down in your liver and turned into glucose. That's why carbohydrates are called "protein sparing"; they spare your protein for being used for energy. And that's why it's ridiculous to go on low-carbohydrate diets to get defined muscles; you will inevitably lose some muscle.

You can always tell when you start using muscle for energy. We pointed out earlier that one pound of muscle tissue contains 600 calories; in contrast, 1 pound of fat contains 3,500 calories. If you were to start burning muscle for energy, how many pounds of muscle would you have to burn in order to get the same energy yield as from a pound of fat? Almost 6 pounds! You will know when you start using muscle for energy because you will start losing weight very rapidly—2 to 5 pounds a day.

The best way to get cut up is to go on a reduced-calorie diet by reducing your daily calorie intake to below your daily maintenance need of calories. If you need 3,000 calories a day to maintain your existing bodyweight and you reduce your daily calorie intake to 2,000 calories, then you're going to be 1,000 calories deficient. Where are those 1,000 calories going to come from? Your bodyfat. That's what bodyfat is—stored energy.

WHY YOU SHOULD STAY LEAN

If you look at a bodybuilder who goes on a zero-carbohydrate diet for a contest, you'll notice a very common phenomenon that happens immediately afterward: He gets fat. It's inevitable because it's a protective mechanism; the body doesn't want to lose all of its bodyfat. As far as the body is concerned, it's starving, it's dying. And it's going to protect itself against this happening again in the future by putting on as much fat as possible. The best thing to do if you desire to stay defined year-round is to get lean slowly over a period of time and then maintain that lower bodyfat level sanely, by eating a well-balanced diet.

There's another reason to stay lean as much of the time as possible. Contrary to what some would have you believe, fat adds nothing in the way of offering an advantage to body strength. In fact, it hinders body strength. It has been discovered that intramuscular fat—that is, fat in between muscle fibers—actually hinders contraction, which serves to make you weaker. The leaner you are, the stronger you'll be.

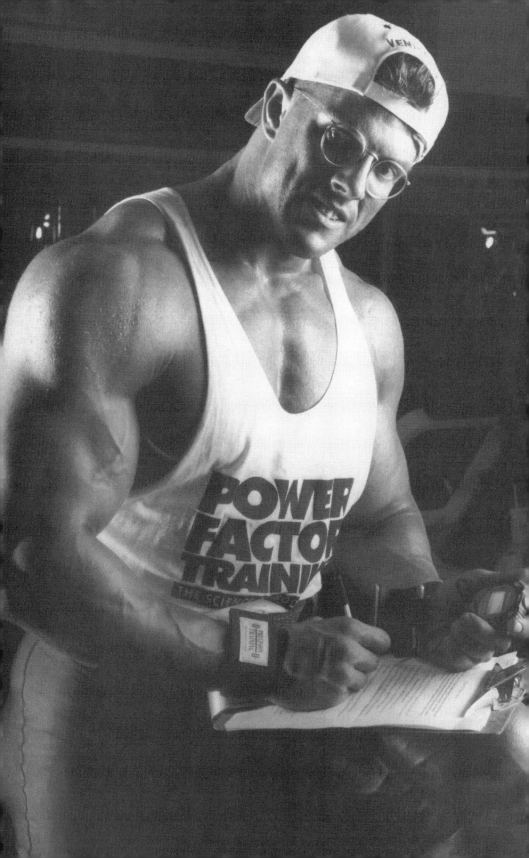

12

Bodybuilding Fact vs. Fiction

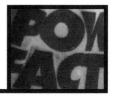

Bodybuilding, as it is commonly practiced, is one of the least scientific endeavors in the sporting world. Not that bodybuilding can't be or is not scientific, but so few individuals have ever taken the time to view it in terms of the related sciences to learn how it ought to be practiced for maximal results.

The simple tools of a pencil and stopwatch are all you need to practice scientific bodybuilding.

GROUNDLESS TRAINING THEORIES

Judging by some of the bizarre and downright fraudulent training beliefs that are currently in vogue these days, as well as by the volume of mail and phone calls we're receiving on a daily basis regarding the Power Factor Training System, it might be safe to say that the time for such a noncontradictory, rational, scientific, and (most importantly) result-producing system of strength training is long overdue. What follows, then, is a look at some of the more prevalent muscle-building beliefs and what basis, if any, a person might have for holding them. The facts of the matter just might surprise you.

Groundless Theory 1: Angle Training Is a Must for Maximum Muscle Development

"You've got to hit the muscle from different angles" is a popular belief these days. Multiple-angle training is predicated on the misconception that by training at different angles, you'll be bringing more muscle fibers into play than would have been activated otherwise. Physiologically, this just isn't the case. More muscle fibers are not brought into play or recruited by changing such comparatively trivial mechanisms as hand spacing or the angle at which you recline your torso. In fact, if you performed an exercise that limited the stress of focus to only one region of a muscle group to the exclusion of all other regions, then, by definition, you would have reduced the potential fiber involvement of the exercise and, hence, its productivity.

The entire argument in support of multiple-angle training as a means of maximizing muscle growth has missed the side of the barn by at least eight yards. The only factor that dictates muscle fiber activation is how heavy the weight is—not the angle through which it's lifted. The heavier the weight, the more fibers are recruited to lift it, meaning that more fibers are stimulated to grow. Even if multiple-angle training could effectively isolate certain sections of a given muscle, it would still be a step in the wrong direction, since limiting the amount of fibers involved in a contraction would reduce the amount receiving growth stimulation.

This is not what any bodybuilder's objective should be. For example, if incline presses could stress only the upper pecs (which they don't), then you would have effectively stimulated only one-third of your pectorals.

You would then have to perform additional pec work to stimulate the remaining two-thirds of your pecs. This is inherently inefficient. All in all, you would have to perform three exercises to stimulate one muscle complex—a monumental waste of time, particularly in light of the fact that both the upper and lower portions of the pec share a common tendon of insertion. The fibers in both regions are activated whenever the muscle complex is called into play.

It doesn't matter to the body whether you train with an incline bench, a decline bench, or a flat bench. For that matter, your muscles can't differentiate between a barbell, a Nautilus machine, or a bucket of rocks. All your muscles are concerned with is whether enough fibers have been recruited to move the resistance you're training with. Since it's your muscle fibers that do all of the lifting, it logically follows that exercises that generate the highest Power Factor and Power Index also involve the most muscle fibers. So train by the numbers, not by preconceived notions regarding multiple inefficient exercises.

Groundless Theory 2: You've Got to "Shock" the Muscle

The belief that you have to shock the muscle in order to make it grow is interesting, if only for its ambiguity. What could this possibly mean? Certainly, if you actually shocked a muscle group, you would have effectively left it incapacitated. Further, if you shocked your muscles and the motor units that supplied them, your entire nervous system would be traumatized—not to mention your cardiac muscle! Remember that muscle has one function and one function only: to contract. That's all a muscle does. That's its sole function. Muscle isn't complicated at all. It's not like the kidneys. Muscle contracts or relaxes. That's it.

If, for example, you decide to shock your biceps muscle by having it perform a curl with a barbell instead of a dumbbell, it still is carrying out its primary function, contraction. So where's the shock? Likewise, if, instead of performing a dumbbell curl sitting up, you perform it lying back on a forty-five-degree angled bench, the action of the biceps muscle is still the same—it contracts. Again, that's its function.

You cannot shock, coax, cajole, or the ever-popular "confuse" a muscle into growth. There's no such thing as a cellular brain in each individual muscle cell that would allow for it to become confused, befuddled, vexed, or filled with any form of angst. Muscle cells receive electrical stimulation from the brain via the central and peripheral nervous systems to either contract or disengage (relax), and that's it.

Groundless Theory 3: Full Range Will Lengthen the Muscles

One of the most prevalent misconceptions in bodybuilding is the belief that a full range of motion will somehow stimulate more muscle fibers near the insertion of a muscle. For example, it was commonly believed that if you performed full-range Preacher curls for your biceps, the stress of the exercise would be more directly focused onto the "lower biceps." This is ridiculous. Fibers, regardless of where they are located in a given muscle, are recruited and hence stimulated by one thing and one thing only: weight.

Muscle fibers are recruited only as needed, meaning if the weight you're attempting to lift has exceeded the capacity of those fibers already activated. Only then will more fibers be activated, and they'll be activated irrespective of what part of the muscle group they happen to reside in. If you want to ensure that all of the available muscle fibers in your biceps will be stimulated to grow bigger and stronger, then you have to employ a resistance that is heavy enough to recruit all available fibers. Excessive stretching and an exaggerated range of motion play no part at all in the process of muscle fiber recruitment.

It just isn't possible to lengthen muscles to any appreciable degree anyway, and certainly not by stretching them. Muscles are attached to bones by tendons, so the only way to lengthen a muscle would be to surgically cut the tendons and reattach them further down the bone. Muscle length is one of those genetic traits that just aren't subject to alteration. So if your biceps aren't as long as Arnold's, forget about it and just focus on developing the best physique you can.

Groundless Theory 4: Isolation Exercises Will Create Definition and Striations

If you ask most bodybuilders, professional or otherwise, why they perform several exercises for a given body part, you'll usually hear a reply something like this: "Well, I perform my basic, heavy, compound movement for size, another movement for shape, and a third to bring out the striations, or quality. Such an answer is absolutely loaded with fallacies. Apart from basic, heavy compound movements for size (they're also the ones that bring out a muscle group's inherent shape, by the way, by virtue of being the ones that stimulate it into growth), there is no such thing as a "shaping" exercise or "definition" movement.

What leads to the creation of definition is the burning of calories beyond what you ingest. The more calories you expend, the greater the likelihood of your becoming defined. Therefore, the exercises that burn the most calories on a per set basis are the ones that will lead to the creation of the greatest definition. And which exercises are these? The same ones you use to build maximum mass: heavy, basic, compound movements. Think about it this way. In which exercise are the weights greatest and the muscular output required to move them the greatest—barbell bench presses with 200 pounds or repping out with a pair of 40-pound dumbbells for a set of flys? Obviously the heavy benches would require far more energy to complete and would generate a higher Power Factor.

As far as striations go, skeletal muscle tissue is striated, and everybody has skeletal muscle tissue. The term *striated* merely refers to the fact that the muscle is arranged longitudinally in bundles. When viewed under a microscope or with the naked eye on a highly defined bodybuilder, muscle striations are clearly visible. There also appears to be a certain genetic predisposition toward striations. For example Mr. Olympia, Dorian Yates, had few striations, whereas a tenth-place finisher, Andreas Munzer, had them everywhere! Certainly, Dorian Yates had every muscle group developed to its maximum on his body. In fact, his muscles were more fully developed than were Munzer's, and certainly both men were at incredibly low bodyfat levels, probably both in the neighborhood of 2 percent—yet Munzer was the one with the striations.

In conclusion, you cannot train for shape or definition more successfully with isolation movements than you can with compound ones, and striations are the result of both an incredibly low percent of bodyfat and a genetic predisposition toward such a condition. They cannot be "trained" into a muscle.

Groundless Theory 5: There's No Such Thing as Overtraining, Only Undereating

One of the more recent misconceptions in bodybuilding regards the issue of overtraining and nutrition. There is no such thing as overtraining, so it goes, only undereating. The implication is that if you overeat, you can accordingly extend the limit to which you can train and, hence, stimulate muscle growth.

This position has absolutely no backing from exercise science. The supply of biochemical resources used up in the process of growth stimulation are limited of necessity and cannot be restored instantaneously, no matter how many calories you consume. Granted, nutrition does affect the degree to which growth can manifest, but to a limited extent. An adequate and optimal intake of nutrients serves to maintain a full supply of the biochemicals utilized in the growth process. Consuming quantities far in excess of that intake does not somehow force the body to expand this supply infinitely.

The body has specific nutritional needs each day, the operative word being *needs*. In the context of nutrition, the term implies a limit that cannot be transcended. It's like a bricklayer who needs exactly 4,000 bricks to build a chimney. He doesn't need 5,000. He doesn't need 4,050. And he doesn't need 4,001. He needs only 4,000 bricks. Likewise with nutrition; the body and its muscles have needs every bit as specific as the bricklayer's (even more so, actually; surplus bricks can be resold or put aside until the next job). Surplus calories—those over and above what's required for maintenance and a little bit extra for the growth you may be stimulating from workout to workout—only result in the deposition of fat.

Therefore, the notion that forced feeding or hyper-nutrition can somehow compensate for the effects of what would otherwise be overtraining simply isn't true. Even at best, muscle growth is negligible on a daily basis anyway. A 30-pound gain of muscle a year—which would be wonderful—averages out to a little more than an ounce a day. An ounce! How many extra calories over and above maintenance levels do you think would be required for such a minuscule amount of growth to manifest? Damn few, obviously. The evidence is that very little extra nutrition beyond what's required for maintenance levels is legitimately needed to gain muscular bodyweight on a consistent basis.

Groundless Theory 6: Train for the Pump, Then You Know You've Stimulated Growth

Many bodybuilders head for the gym with the idea that getting a good pump is the key to muscle growth stimulation. Unfortunately, there exists no evidence whatsoever that a pump is an index of muscle growth stimulation. All bodybuilders achieve a pump to some degree every time they work out, yet, obviously, not all bodybuilders grow as a result of each workout. For that matter, people who perform high-volume exercise, such as cyclists, joggers, and even StairMaster enthusiasts, also experience a pump but don't experience growth as a result. If the pump was the sine qua non of muscle growth stimulation, then all of the aforementioned athletes would be jumping up in weight classes on an almost weekly basis. A pump is simply edema, or the temporary swelling of tissue due to a buildup of fluid—in this case blood—in the muscle being worked. Unless growth was stimulated as a result of a workout, however, the muscle will revert to its previous size once the pump subsides.

Strength training, which is what proper bodybuilding really is, doesn't always produce much in the way of a pump. Still, there can be no mistaking the fact that, after a hard peak-overload workout, the body is about to undergo some profound physiological changes. Increase your rate of work, or Power Factor, and your muscles *will get stronger.*

And therein lies the key to muscle growth. It was discovered a long, long time ago that muscular size and strength are directly related. More precisely, the strength of a muscle is proportional to its cross-sectional area. In other words, a stronger muscle is a bigger muscle. That's why when you remove a limb that's been immobilized due to injury from a cast, you notice that it's atrophied or become smaller from disuse. What's the doctor's prescription for rehabilitating that limb? To get those muscles to grow bigger again? Strength training! And the stronger the limb becomes, the bigger it becomes.

Such is the nature of the relationship between size and strength, and it couldn't be otherwise. Could you, for example, imagine a massively muscled bodybuilder like Paul DeMayo being able to bench-press only 100 pounds? No, Paul works out with over 400 pounds on the bench press, and he has the muscles to prove it. In other words, Paul is as big as he is because he is as strong as he is.

If you want to grow bigger and bigger muscles, you should always train with an eye toward a strength improvement, as reflected in your Power Factor and Power Index. A pump, while a nice feeling admittedly, is not an accurate indicator of muscle growth stimulation.

Groundless Theory 7: Plyometrics
Another popular theory in training these days is that of plyometrics. This postulates that if you take a moderate weight but use explosive, fast repetitions, you'll stimulate only the fast-twitch muscle fibers. This is yet another bit of fiction. Muscle fibers are recruited in an orderly fashion according to the resistance level they're being called upon to move. What recruits the fast-twitch fibers is the heaviness of the weight to be lifted (or, more specifically, its force requirements) and not, as the plyometric advocates would have you believe, the speed at which you perform the movement.

For you to move a weight quickly, it must be light, because the lighter the weight, the quicker you can move it. Moving a light weight, however, irrespective of the velocity at which you move it, only requires slow-twitch fibers. Demands of low muscular intensity are always met by the slow-twitch fibers. Intermediate fibers come into play once the slow-twitch fibers are no longer able to continue the task. The fast-twitch fibers—the ones with the greatest mass potential—are finally recruited when the other two sets of fibers can no longer meet the force requirements. Therefore, when the fast-twitch fibers are activated, all fibers are activated, including the slow- and intermediate-twitch. And again, this recruitment process depends not on velocity but on force, the amount of force required to move the weight. The heaviest weights require the greatest force and, hence, recruitment of fibers.

Plyometric movements, with the light to moderate weights employed, cannot activate fast-twitch fibers. There simply is no evidence that movements performed in an explosive or ballistic fashion will—magically—bypass the slow and intermediate fibers in order to recruit solely fast-twitch fibers. There is, however, ample evidence that jumping and bouncing while holding heavy weights will cause injuries.

Groundless Theory 8: Full-Range Squats Are the Best Exercise Ever!

Mark Berry and Perry Reader wrote volumes in the 1930s and '40s about the "wondrous, overall muscle-building benefits of full squats." These beliefs have persisted to this day—and not without reason. According to men like the Readers (editors of *Ironman Magazine*), who contributed much to the iron game, squats had a stimulating effect on the entire system. They were right. Performing full-range squats, although a weak-range exercise, did and will stimulate phenomenal overall muscle growth—simply because the amount of weight (overload) utilized in full-range squats is superior to the weight utilized in any other weak-range movement. It wasn't the squats per se that stimulated this wondrous overall growth, but rather the fact that squats were the vehicle for using heavy weights to tax the central nervous system enough to cause an adaptive response. An even greater demand would have been placed on the CNS by the performance of strongest-range squats, for the very same reason—heavier weights could have been employed.

Quarter squats would not only have produced greater muscle growth stimulation but would have been much safer as well. Besides causing excessive shear forces in the knee joint, full-range squats cause severe compression of the spinal column, particularly in the bottom position, where the anterior aspect of the lumbar vertebrae is compressed. What happens is that the intervertebral discs end up getting pushed backward, which could result in either herniated or ruptured discs. Research has consistently revealed electromyographic activity of up to ten times bodyweight in the lumbar region when full squats are performed with as little as an individual's bodyweight. So while squatting may be a very productive exercise, if not *the* most productive exercise, full squats are definitely not the way to go.

Groundless Theory 9: Pre-Exhaustion

No matter how much a muscle is used, it will not grow larger or stronger until it is overloaded. This means that the intensity of the work required of it must be increased above what it is currently accustomed to performing. That is, the muscle must be required to exert more power or work against a greater resistance than before. According to exercise physiologists (who make their careers out of studying closely the cause-and-effect relationships of such things), hypertrophy, or the increase in the cross-sectional area of a muscle's fibers, can best be triggered by increasing both the amount of weight lifted (overload) and the rate of work or pounds lifted per minute (the Power Factor). The higher the overload and rate of work, the greater the adaptive response of muscle growth. It is the central nervous system that triggers the growth process, which cannot be called into play by the isolated and protracted performance of highly repetitive tasks that are of a level well within the body's existing muscular capacity.

The fact is that growth is systemic, and the trigger mechanism that signals the body to grow can only be turned on by a call to arms from the central nervous system. Growth isn't easy; it must literally be forced to occur. Such being the case, how does one force growth with light weights or mild exertion? The answer is, one can't— at least not without growth drugs.

Taking the preceding facts into consideration, it becomes much easier to evaluate all training methodologies, including one that gained a tremendous amount of exposure and popularity during the 1970s—the pre-exhaustion principle. Pre-exhaustion became so popular that Arthur Jones, the much-heralded creator of Nautilus exercise equipment, designed several of his machines with an isolation/compound component built into them to take full advantage of it. For the sake of illustration, pre-exhaustion requires that an isolation movement be performed prior to a compound movement with literally zero rest time between the two.

The fact that isolation movements necessitate that lighter weights be used than would be utilized for compound movements is enough of an indicator to tell you that this system is heading in the wrong direction. Second, if it's a full-range isolation movement, the weights are reduced even further. Therefore your muscles are performing less work (moving less weight) over a given unit of time—per set. That's just for openers. When the compound movement is performed immediately after the isolation movement, the resistance must also be reduced in order for the temporarily fatigued muscles to continue to contract. Usually this resistance is in the neighborhood of 50 percent less than what the trainee would normally use. Again, a reduced resistance.

Given that the clinical formula for hypertrophy is increased work in a unit of time, pre-exhaust is a step towards doing *less* work, *less* total weight lifted in a unit of time. Sure, you're doing two sets back to back, but with lighter weight. Additionally, the reps performed in pre-exhaust total out to roughly 6 to 8 per set, which is a total of 12 to 16, or roughly half the amount of reps performed in one strong-range set—with much less resistance. The result? Little or no muscle growth.

Granted, muscle can be stimulated to grow using methods such as pre-exhaustion, but only minimally. Maximal stimulation cannot be obtained with such a system, because it calls for such a reduced level of muscular output.

According to the law of muscle fiber recruitment, the heavier the weight, the more muscle fibers are called into play to move it. Conversely, the lighter the weight, the fewer fibers that are required to move it. The pre-exhaustion system incorporates lighter weights and reduced muscular overload, so it is not nearly as efficient a muscle-building system as some advocates might have initially believed.

Groundless Theory 10: Instinctive Training

A very loud school in bodybuilding advocates that you must "trust your instincts," as opposed to science, when it comes to building muscles. "Go with your gut," say the advocates of this theory, called instinctive training. The funny thing is that they actually mean it!

Never in his wildest dreams (and some of them were pretty wild indeed) would Sigmund Freud, the father of modern psychiatry, have ever postulated that our species has a "bodybuilding instinct." An instinct to build big muscles in order to ultimately rub baby oil on them and go up on a stage and pose? It's downright laughable. Even if such an instinct did exist (and we by no means grant the premise of man being an instinctive creature), attempting to monitor your results by such a subjective index as how you felt at any given time would, in the final analysis, yield you nothing. I could feel that I was having the greatest workout of my life, but if my Power Factor and Power Index were down, I'd be grossly mistaken.

Only in bodybuilding could one postulate such a ludicrous theory as instinctive training and get away with it. Could you imagine, for example, an Olympic sprinter trying to monitor his progress by "feel" or "instinct"? Of his never having measured his progress by using a stopwatch? Or of never having any tangible, objective measure of the effects of his training techniques nor of his improvement from one month to the next? Yet this is exactly the kind of irrational, low-tech methodology that bodybuilders have always used.

Until Power Factor Training came on the scene, no objective gauges by which to accurately measure one's progress or lack thereof had ever been applied to bodybuilding. Power Factor Training allows bodybuilders to measure and find the optimum point where they can sustain their highest workload or Power Factor and, hence, their greatest degree of muscle growth stimulation—the effectiveness of which shows up in their workout numbers.

Feeling something to be true is no guarantee that it is true. Boeing Aircraft doesn't employ individuals who simply have "a good feeling about aerodynamics" to design their airplanes; they hire people with bona fide scientific backgrounds who understand and can objectively measure the parameters of safe, efficient aircraft. And so it is in any endeavor involving science, including bodybuilding. Or at least it should be. After all, it was science, not instinct, that sent men to the moon, cured disease, controlled the environment, and determined how muscle growth is really stimulated.

THE FACTS ABOUT SUPPLEMENTS

One of the biggest concerns facing the bodybuilder of the nineties is the role of supplements. Never before has such an emphasis been placed on nutrition. Unfortunately, it is this very aspect of bodybuilding that is the most neglected. A contradiction? No, only an apparent one. Remember that supplements and nutrition are two entirely different things. Nutrition is what we obtain daily from the foods we eat. Supplements, on the other hand, are only a factor when we're unable to obtain the nutrition our bodies require from those same foods. Supplements do play a role in nutrition when they're used as the term implies—supplementally.

The single most important fact regarding nutrition for the bodybuilder, athlete, bowler, homemaker, or anyone else who wishes to maintain health and build a strong body is the unequivocal need for a well-balanced diet. A sound diet is one that daily provides all the nutrients—protein, carbs, fats, vitamins, minerals, and water—necessary for maintaining health. Ironically, bodybuilders often forget that bodily health is the first requisite for building a muscular physique.

When you are unable to maintain a well-balanced diet, or if you suspect that you're deficient in a particular nutrient, *then* and only then can a case be made for resorting to protein powders, carb drinks, and vitamin/ mineral supplements. Remember, supplements were never intended to be used as foods or to replace them in the diet. When this has happened in the past, such as when liquid protein diets were voguish back in the seventies, several deaths resulted. Again, supplements can only be justified when used supplementally, when particular deficiencies exist and can't be redressed by a closer attention to diet.

For example, bodybuilders who diet severely for a contest must be especially careful because reduced-calorie diets are often so restrictive that the body does not receive many essential nutrients. Most nutritional scientists agree that a well-balanced diet becomes impossible once your daily caloric consumption drops below 1,500 calories per day. However, barring such conditions, the only things supplements represent is a lack of attention to one's food selection and meal preparation. That and a colossal waste of money.

Amino Acids
It's absolutely amazing just how many bodybuilders readily accept the notion that amino acid supplements are somehow a primary requisite in the muscle growth process. The history of amino acid supplements can be traced to a few years back, when protein supplements became for a time rather unpopular with the bodybuilding community. Scientific information then being disseminated by biochemists, physiologists, and nutritionally informed bodybuilders, such as Mike Mentzer, insisted that a well-balanced diet provided more than enough protein for the aspiring bodybuilder and that supplements were, by and large, simply a waste of money and the body's energy in digesting them. At this point, the protein manufacturers, in an attempt to recapture the tremendously lucrative protein market, reissued the protein supplements—only this time with a new name, "amino acids." It's another example of old wine in new skins. Amino acids are simply the nitrogen-based constituents of protein

and, consequently, yield the same effect as their soya, milk, egg, and beef predecessors.

Of course, not only did the labels change but also the marketing strategies employed to promote the "new" products. Amino acid supplements were now accompanied by ad campaigns declaring that they were actually safe, effective, and even superior replacements to anabolic steroids. That is tantamount to telling a man who is testosterone deficient that all he needs is a good protein shake in order to set things right. It is at once obvious that such claims were ludicrous; after all, protein is a nutritional element, whereas a steroid is a hormone. There exists no similarity between the two at all. One is a dietary constituent, while the other is a drug—and that's a big difference.

Of course, amino acids are absolutely necessary for proper bodily and muscular function, including muscle growth. But it makes no difference at all to your body whether they're in the form of a capsule, a pill, or a T-bone steak. Your body simply breaks down the macromolecule of protein into its constituent amino acids and redistributes the individual amino acids to where they're needed most. However, unlike the sugars that enter the blood from carbohydrates, each amino acid retains its distinctive chemical structure in order to be utilized to make up the varied sequences and structures of human proteins.

The body has specific needs for protein; additional amounts, such as those obtained through supplements, serve no biological value. As long as the cells have all the amino acids they need, additional amino acids (regardless of how they were consumed) will not be put to work. Making more amino acids available will not make cells multiply or renew at a faster rate. In fact, pouring excess amino acids into your body is no different than giving a contractor more lumber than he needs to build a house.

The genes that shape our bodies—and particularly our muscular development—provide each cell with instructions for making proteins from amino acids. These instructions must be precise. A small change in amino acid sequence or structure can make a protein unusable—or even lethal. The method by which the trillions of cells in the human body encode and use this information has been known since 1962, when James Watson, Francis Crick, and Maurice Wilkins discovered how the instructions for making the more than 100,000 proteins of the body were carried in every cell by a tiny amount of DNA—a discovery for which they were awarded the Nobel Prize that same year.

These cells determine what proteins have to be made and then signal the chromosomes in the nucleus that a specific protein is needed. DNA itself is a chain of nucleotides, each of which is made of sugar, a phosphate, and a base. It's the sequencing of the nucleotides in DNA that actually instructs the cells in how to make the various proteins that the body needs. The DNA nucleotides are partly made from a sugar called deoxyribose, from which DNA (deoxyribonucleic acid) takes its name. The free-floating nucleotides are made with the sugar ribose; the chains that they eventually make up are known as ribonucleic acids, or RNA.

Because RNA relentlessly seeks out only amino acids, and because we know that all molecules of any one amino acid are completely interchangeable, we can conclude that for protein synthesis the food source of the amino acids does not matter. For example, if the amino acid lysine is what the DNA blueprint calls for, the transfer RNA will seek lysine and nothing else, without concern for whether that lysine molecule comes from a hot dog, a can of tuna, sunflower seeds, soy sprouts, or an amino acid supplement. Further, lysine from one source cannot be different from that of any other; if it were, it could not be used.

There is evidence that we really do much better when the amino acids come from foods as opposed to supplements. Apparently, the complicated mechanisms of absorbing amino acids from the intestine require that some amino acid chains be present. When attempting to maintain the nutrition of the ill, especially those who have digestive problems (such as postsurgical patients), physicians have found that pure amino acids taken by mouth are not that well absorbed. When liquid foods (which are used for patients) are formulated with a mix of some pure amino acids and short chains, there seems to be better absorption.

Again, amino acids are not a requisite for building big muscles. To build big muscles, you must first stimulate muscle growth at the cellular level via peak-overload training and then allow sufficient time to elapse between workouts in order to allow your muscular reserves time to recover and grow. Then and only then does nutrition become a factor in the growth process.

Adequate nutrition of all nutrients, not just protein or amino acids, must be provided in order for you to maintain your existing level of muscle mass. If you stimulated growth by training with sufficient overload, you must consume a little bit extra (approximately 16 calories, including 0.9 gram of protein per kilogram of bodyweight) in order to allow that growth to manifest. To get adequate nutrition, you simply need a well-balanced diet. Such a diet includes six to eleven portions of cereals and grains; two to five portions of fruits and vegetables; two to three portions of meats, fish, and poultry; and two to three portions of dairy products each day. These will provide you with sufficient nutrition to maintain your health and, if you've stimulated it, allow for the growth of additional muscle mass.

In sum, there is no way that amino acid supplements can by themselves either stimulate or accelerate the muscle growth process.

RETHINKING PERIODIZATION

Much has been written in the muscle magazines recently about the importance of "periodization" or "cycling" your workout routines throughout the course of a year. The authors of the pro-periodization articles liken bodybuilding to architecture. "You can't build a house without a blueprint," they preach, "so you've got to map out your training plans accordingly." It's a cute metaphor admittedly, although somewhat incongruous.

After all, it would be an odd—and infrequently employed—architect indeed who would propose dividing up the construction of a house into "seasons." Not to mention the fact that muscle cells are living organisms, not composed of pine and drywall, and therefore cannot be treated as such. As I said, it was a cute metaphor, just not a very practical one.

As far as the concept of periodization itself is concerned, its advocates maintain that certain months of the year (or cycles) should be set aside for training with different weights, reps, and, in some instances, goals, which its proponents tell you ahead of time are required for ultimate success. The truth, however, is that there exists no reason for periodization, particularly if you are a "clean" athlete (one who doesn't use steroids). The concept of periodization was created by the Russian Olympic lifting coaches in an attempt to synchronize the lifting of heavy weights with their lifters' drug cycles (hence the term *cycling*). When they were on steroids and growth hormones, they were stronger and able to train much harder and heavier than they were when they were off the drugs. As a result, periods of heavy lifting were structured to coincide with their drug cycles and then periods of lighter, less intense lifting were introduced into the schedule to reduce the chance of burnout and injury as the athletes came off the drugs. When the Soviet lifters were winning titles, an American coach inquired about their "training system" and was told that they "divided the routines up into periods of heavy lifting along with periods of not-so-heavy lifting." In a perfect textbook example of the fallacy *Post hoc, ergo propter hoc,* the U.S. coach assumed that because their success came after following this cycling system, it had to be the *result* of following this system. From this was born the entire periodization concept, complete with its "Muscle Refinement Phase."

If you really want for a day's work sometime, try to look up this term in any muscle physiology textbook. Why do I say this? Simply because it doesn't exist. You can do one of three things with muscle tissue: maintain its size, increase its size (hypertrophy), or decrease its size (atrophy). A bodybuilder seeking to increase his muscle size must first train hard enough to stimulate growth and then rest long enough between workouts to allow that growth to manifest. It's as simple as that. After all, this isn't crude oil we're dealing with, it's muscle tissue and therefore not subject to any process of "refinement." Muscle has one function: it contracts. And when it contracts against resistance that is increased on a progressive basis, it grows bigger and stronger.

Quite apart from the fact that the entire periodization concept is based on a misconception is the fact that there's simply no evidence that engaging in activities that have been shown to have no effect on the process of muscle growth (such as training with lighter weights and reduced muscular output) will, if it's "structured properly," somehow hasten the muscle growth process. And what if you're feeling strong as a bull when you head for the gym and know you're capable of really setting some personal best records that day, but it's the "Refinement Phase" you happen to be in this month, not the "Maximum Mass Phase," so you have to pull back on the throttle this workout? How does such gibberish result in anything except spinning your wheels and reduced progress? The clinical formula for muscle growth is increased work (overload) over a unit of time. Anything other than this will not stimulate muscle growth—period.

EXERCISE: HOW LITTLE YOU NEED!

Heavy-overload exercise—the only kind that results in immediate muscular adaptation—is a form of stress to the muscles and the overall physical system. When performed properly, such training will stimulate a compensatory buildup in the form of additional muscle size and strength, which aids the body in coping more successfully with similar stressors in the future. However, bodybuilders who insist on training six to seven days a week (on a system of three days on, one day off or four days on, one day off) will witness a decompensatory effect. The resulting drain on the regulatory subsystems of the body will actually prevent the buildup of muscle tissue. In fact, the body will have to call on all of its energy reserves simply to attempt to overcome the energy debt caused by such overtraining.

These facts strongly indicate that the less time spent in the gym, the better your results will be. You'll find that your results will be spectacular if you limit your total training time to one, two, or—at the most—three workouts per week of roughly forty-five to sixty minutes per session.

Although recovery time will vary from individual to individual, most people starting out require a bare minimum of forty-eight hours between workouts in order to recover and grow stronger. As the trainee grows stronger, the less training his body will be able to handle before becoming overtrained and catabolic. When you use Power Factor Training, you will be able to see the extent to which you have recovered by virtue of your Power Factor and Power Index numbers. If you return to the gym too soon after a workout, you will not perform as well, and your numbers will reflect this. When this happens, just add a day or two of recovery until your numbers show some improvement.

Like all other physical characteristics of humans, the time needed between workouts in order for complete recovery and growth to manifest will vary widely among individuals. After identical workouts, one person may be able to return to the gym in forty-eight hours and see an increase in his Power Factor and Power Index. Another person may need as many as eight weeks to go by in order to recover sufficiently and show improvement.

Hard to believe, you say? Consider that the May 1993 issue of the *Journal of Physiology* reported that a group of men and women aged twenty-two to thirty-two took part in an exercise experiment in which they trained their forearms in a negative-only fashion to a point of muscular failure. Negatives are considered by some exercise physiologists to be more important than positive or concentric contractions, because more weight can be employed. In any event, all of the subjects agreed that they were most sore two days after exercising and that the soreness was gone by the ninth day. But it took most of the people nearly six weeks to regain just half of the strength they had before the workout! The experimenters concluded that muscles are drained far more severely by intense exercise than was previously thought. According to this research, the muscles of some individuals can literally take months to heal and adapt after an intensive workout.

It is clear that the spacing of workouts, then, can be measured along a range of time. That range begins with the first day you can return to the gym and expect to see an improvement, and it ends with the last day you can return to the gym and expect to see an improvement. Power Factor Training will allow you to precisely determine your personal range of recovery ability, which—depending on a variety of personal factors—may be anywhere from a few days to many weeks.

Regardless of what your personal range of recovery happens to be, one thing is for certain: Everyone's personal recovery ability takes much longer to complete itself than was initially thought. Training more than three days a week—and maybe even once a week—is a mistake for most bodybuilders who are looking to increase their muscle mass.

THE FACTS ABOUT STEROIDS

To state, as some bodybuilders do, that steroids only add perhaps 10 percent of polish to one's physique may be the biggest joke in professional bodybuilding. It's unfortunately more like 90 percent of everything you see. This is unsettling for a number of reasons, not the least of which is the fact that these drugs are illegal. Beyond that, however, is the fact that if bodybuilders can get their results out of a pill or bottle, then they have no vested interest in trying to determine just what kind of progress can be made without the drugs.

It's a medical fact that if you take large quantities of anabolic steroids and don't train, your muscles will not grow. However, your muscles *will* grow if you train with a large quantity of muscular output and don't take any anabolic steroids. Granted, if you take anabolic steroids and train properly, your muscles will grow even larger, but these facts do show that training, not drugs, is the key to turning on the muscle growth process. This was verified by studies conducted at Harvard University over twenty years ago in which Alfred Goldberg and his colleagues discovered that if adequate stimulation is present, muscle tissue will grow. Further, they noted that it will grow quickly and in proportion to the severity of the stimulation and in the absence of influences such as testosterone, growth hormone, insulin, and even food! Stimulation, then, is the first requisite. Steroids play a secondary role in the muscle growth process.

Yes, they do work, but it gives pause for thought that, if the right kind of stimulation is present, muscle will grow and continue to grow if that stimulation remains present. No bodybuilder has yet trained over an entire career with a precise means of monitoring his results to ensure that such a level of stimulation was present. It therefore remains to be seen what the ultimate limits truly are for the drug-free human body.

THE SEVEN MYTHS OF BODYBUILDING

Myth 1: Big Muscles Will Slow You Down

Many coaches and personal trainers believe that an increase in the size and strength of a muscle will result in slower movements when performing a particular athletic event. Boxing, for example, always maintained that weight training would slow down the punching speed of the boxer. However, just the opposite takes place. The speed at which you can perform a particular movement will be enhanced tremendously by increasing your strength levels. The speed of a body movement depends on two factors: (1) the strength of the muscles that are actually involved when performing a specific skill and (2) your capacity to recruit muscle fibers while performing the movement (neurological efficiency).

It's fallacious to assume that a muscle will "slow down" because of an increase in its strength and size. The correlation between the speed of a muscle movement and the strength level of the muscle is positive. Therefore, to increase the speed of a muscle movement, increase the strength of the muscles needed to perform that particular movement.

Myth 2: All That Muscle Turns to Fat Eventually
Perhaps the most common misconception in bodybuilding (particularly to the nonbodybuilder) is that the muscle you build will eventually turn to fat. That belief is totally divorced from reality. Muscle can no more be turned into fat than an apple can be turned into an orange. They are two entirely different cells; one cannot magically become the other.

If you were to chemically analyze fat and muscle, you would discover that muscle and fat both contain varying amounts of protein, water, lipids, and inorganic materials. However, when muscle is exercised, it contracts and produces movement, whereas fat will not contract and is usually stored in the body as a source of fuel. It is physiologically and chemically impossible to convert a muscle to fat and vice versa.

A simple explanation of what takes place can be illustrated by observing the ex-athlete's pattern of exercise and caloric intake. When an athlete stops training his or her muscles, the muscles will begin to atrophy, or shrink from disuse. At the same time, the athlete may continue to consume the same level of calories. With the athlete consuming more calories than are needed to maintain his or her bodyweight and energy demands, the excess is stored in the body as additional fat. If an athlete becomes obese after terminating a strength-training program, it is due to caloric imbalance—taking in more than he's burning off—and not muscle transforming to fat.

Some individuals believe that their bodyweight should maintain a constant level upon the termination of a strength-training program. Unfortunately, these individuals fail to understand that if they lose ten pounds of muscle mass through muscle atrophy and their body weight remains the same, then the weight loss that is attributed to muscle atrophy has been replaced by deposits of additional fat. Thus, if you stop training, you should also reduce your calorie intake.

Myth 3: Lifting Heavy Weights Is Bad for the Joints

Some people worry that they will injure their joints if they lift heavy weights. However, the term *heavy* is relative—heavy compared to what? Nothing can be evaluated without standards for comparison. And, in Power Factor Training, the only person whose standards are significant for making comparisons is yourself.

More to the point, Power Factor Training, properly using what for you are considered "heavy" weights, will actually strengthen the muscles that surround each joint. This, in turn, makes the joint more stable and less susceptible to injury. In fact, proper overload on the ligaments and tendons in the joint region actually serves to thicken them (much as a callous forms on the hands), making them far stronger than they ordinarily would be.

Such a practice must, however, be undertaken cautiously. A greater potential for injury lies not in performing heavy strongest-range training movements (which are within the body's most advantageous leverage and muscular range) but in full-range movements that put the joints and connective tissues in their weakest position, thereby exceeding (often considerably) the structural integrity of the joints and connective tissues. Extreme stretching of joints can, in fact, cause very real damage to ligaments and tendons.

Myth 4: You Train with Heavy Weights and Low Reps for Mass and Light Weights and High Reps for Definition

Despite what some trainers will tell you, there is no magic number of reps to perform for building mass or increasing definition. Remember that muscular definition is primarily the result of dieting off subcutaneous fat so that the muscles directly beneath the skin appear in bold relief. To accelerate the arrival of such a degree of definition, you really don't have to train with weights at all. Running even a mile a day will burn far and away more calories than would the performance of an extra set of bench presses or cable crossovers.

In any event, it is well substantiated that training with peak overload causes the greatest adaptive response by the CNS. As long as you're training with your highest possible Power Index, you will have done all you reasonably can to stimulate an adaptive increase in your muscle mass stores.

Myth 5: You Have to Work a Muscle Through a Full Range of Motion in Order to Fully Develop It

Nowhere has there ever been a study that stated that a full range of motion is a requisite to stimulating maximum muscle growth. The contention of some that partial or strongest-range movements aren't as effective as full-range movements because you're only lifting the weight a few inches is totally unsupported by science.

The truth of the matter is that muscle fiber recruitment (and, therefore, growth stimulation) is a matter of force requirements, not flexibility. The range of motion therefore is not a factor in the muscle growth process. If it were, yoga masters and contortionists would be the most muscularly massive individuals on the planet.

In other words, if you can lift heavier weight, you will recruit more muscle fibers—regardless of the range you use to lift it. The body isn't concerned about such aesthetic factors as whether or not your biceps have extended all the way down on a Preacher curl. In fact, in terms of its energy systems, the body can't tell if you're training your quads or your pecs; its sole concern is how much energy and fiber recruitment are required to move that tremendously heavy weight at the end of your arms.

When your muscles have suddenly been called upon to lift a very heavy weight for a lot of repetitions, a tremendous amount of energy must be created—quickly. The body, then, concerns itself with factors such as muscle fiber activation, hormone secretion, increased blood flow to the working muscles, clearing waste by-products as quickly as possible, initiating the Krebs cycle, and a host of other metabolic activities. With strongest-range training, the two requirements for inducing hypertrophy (maximal overload and increased work in a unit of time) are brought to bear on the skeletal muscles in a manner that no other training method can even remotely approximate.

Myth 6: Real Gains in Mass and Strength Will Come When You Learn How to "Feel" the Exercises You Perform and Train "Instinctively"

The issue as to whether or not man is an instinctual creature is best left to the realm of philosophy and psychology. However, to postulate that man, somewhere in the innermost recesses of his psyche, possesses some sort of a "bodybuilding instinct" or "training instinct" is downright ludicrous.

Even if such a thing did exist, attempting to monitor one's results by such a subjective index as how you felt at any given time would be tantamount to having no way of monitoring one's results. Can you envision an athlete in any other sport engaging in his training in such a haphazard and subjective fashion? Could you imagine, for example, an Olympic miler trying to monitor his progress by feel or instinct and never measuring his progress with a stopwatch? Yet this is exactly the type of irrational, low-tech methodology that bodybuilders have always used. There has always been a technological barrier to finding out the validity of training beliefs and methodologies.

No objective gauges by which to accurately measure one's progress or lack thereof have ever been applied to the sport. In their place are maxims such as "no pain, no gain," "high reps for definition, low reps for mass," "incline presses for your upper pecs," and "muscle confusion," with no objective method to measure their efficacy. What makes Power Factor Training revolutionary is its ability to measure and find the optimum point where you can sustain your highest Power Factor (and, hence, greatest degree of muscle growth stimulation) while accumulating your highest total weight. This is achieved by determining the best combination of weights, reps, and sets for each exercise that you perform. Results can then be simply calculated and even graphed to immediately reveal the effectiveness of your workout. This newfound technology negates the need for cookie-cutter routines that prescribe predetermined numbers of sets, reps, and weights irrespective of the tremendous physical and physiological variation among athletes.

Myth 7: Never Train Less than Three Days per Week, or Your Muscles Will Get Smaller

The issue of training frequency still is cause for debate among individuals (including supposed authorities) in the realm of bodybuilding. Even solid writers such as Arthur Jones and Ellington Darden, Ph.D., who have injected liberal doses of much-needed sanity into the realm of bodybuilding, still have some unwarranted suppositions (and not a little dogma) in their conclusions. One of these areas is in the realm of training frequency.

Darden writes that a three-day-per-week routine is best regardless of your level of development: "A first workout is performed on Monday, a second on Wednesday, and a third on Friday. On Sunday your body is expecting and is prepared for a fourth workout, but it doesn't come."[1] What exactly is this? Certainly not science. The biceps muscles don't talk to the triceps muscles midway through Sunday afternoon and say, "Wasn't there supposed to be a workout today? I was kind of expecting a workout today. I mean, it's been forty-eight hours, and we had one forty-eight hours ago."

To our knowledge, there is nothing in the scientific literature to suggest that muscle tissue thinks (despite the misapplied term of *muscle memory* to the condition of reconditioning an atrophied muscle) by any manner or means. Muscle tissue, you'll be pleased to note, is wonderfully uncomplicated. Muscle tissue will do one of three things: atrophy (from disuse), hypertrophy (from overload training and rest), or remain the same (from genetics and mild stimulation). Technically, muscle action is even more simple; muscles either contract or relax, depending on the neural impulse they receive. It's that simple.

Rather than waste time trying to outwit nonthinking tissue into growing bigger and stronger, the simple solution to building muscle, once you've stimulated growth through heavy overload training, is simply to take adequate time off between workouts to recover and allow the growth you may have stimulated to manifest. Your Power Factor and Power Index numbers will instantly reveal to you whether or not you need more time off. If your numbers are increasing, you're doing fine and your frequency of training is perfect. If they're decreasing, you haven't allowed enough time for recovery and growth to take place. Trying to pigeonhole your physiology into responding to a three-day-per-week program—once it's obvious that you're no longer gaining on such a system— simply because Arthur Jones at one time believed this to be the best way to space out workouts is tantamount to no reasoning whatsoever.

Much of the confusion regarding training frequency might arise from the fact that bodybuilders misunderstand the low-intensity, low-muscular-output feeling of aerobics (which is highly repetitive, daily activity), which causes some pumping or edema of tissue (the same way lifting heavy weights does) but is perceived by the body and the central nervous system as a very low intensity activity. And rightly so. However, while it's true that you can stand literally hours and hours of daily low-intensity activity, the same cannot be said of high-intensity, maximum-overload activity, which is the kind necessary to stimulate maximum gains in muscle mass. It's a case of apples and oranges. Power Factor Training is not aerobics or yoga, so the recovery periods following a Power Factor Training workout must be protracted simply to allow the growth you've stimulated to take place.

Incidentally, in some of his more recent writings, Arthur Jones has advanced the notion that training three times per week is probably less effective than training once a week would be. He's drawn this conclusion based on his own empirical observations and some carefully considered conclusions. But then, it was never Jones who was all that dogmatic about his conclusions, but rather his followers. Jones, to my recollection, always stated that his research was a paradigm until contrary evidence proved it outdated or incorrect.

Nevertheless, any claim to truth without evidence or data cited to back it up is simply predicated on the logical fallacy of "appeal to authority." When unwarranted claims supersede all else—even empirical evidence to the contrary—such information ceases to become science (which is always amenable to reason or evidence). Science, if it is to be truly an intellectual movement, cannot be planned by any central authority; it has to be open to refinement and extension. Once it becomes a closed system, impervious to research or modification, it ceases to be science and becomes, instead, dogma.

In conclusion, you don't need to "shock" or "confuse" your muscle cells to get them to grow bigger and stronger. You simply have to subject them to progressive overload and give them adequate rest afterward.

NOTE

1. Ellington Darden, *100 High-Intensity Ways to Improve Your Bodybuilding* (New York: Pedigree Books, 1989), 161–62.

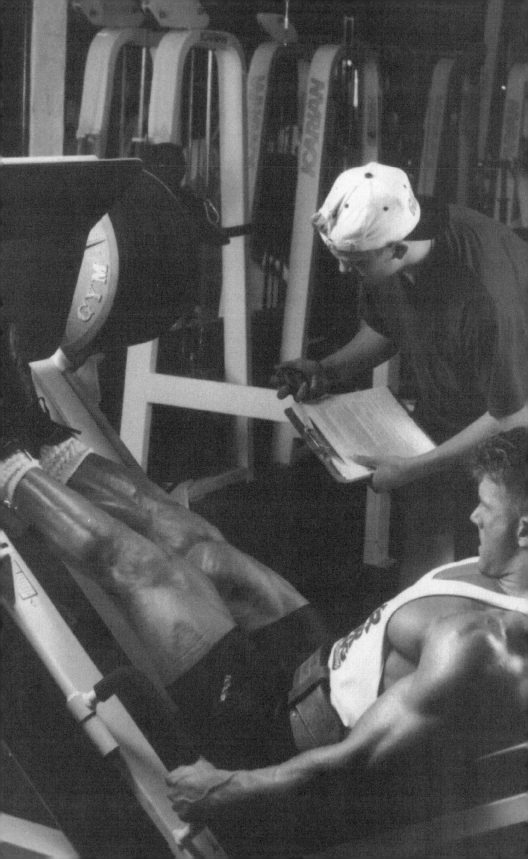

13

Questions and Answers

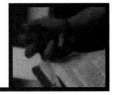

PERIODIZATION

Q: Much has been written in the muscle and powerlifting magazines recently about the importance of
cycling your workout routines to prevent overtraining. They say that you have to do this in order
to stress the muscles differently and shock the muscles back into growing again. They also advise that
doing so gives the body a break from heavy workouts, which, according to them, lead rapidly to overtraining. What is Power Factor Training's response
to this?

A: The Power Factor Training response is the same
as that of enlightened exercise physiologists. We
reject the theory of cycling or periodization,
wherein you reduce intensity in favor of increasing
the duration and frequency of workouts, which is
postulated as a method for building muscular mass
and strength. There is simply no evidence that
engaging in activities that have been shown to have

*Train by the
numbers, and
everything else
will look after
itself.*

no effect on the process of hypertrophy will, if they're scheduled a certain way, somehow enhance the hypertrophy process.

People who advocate the "need" for periodization are ignoring the fact that muscular overload must be progressive in order to trigger adaptation. For example, if you are capable of lifting 5,000 pounds per minute in your bench press routine, what would be the point of several weeks or months of lifting 3,000 pounds per minute? How could that possibly trigger growth?

A properly conducted Power Factor Training routine also compensates for the stress on the body because it's carried on only for brief periods and includes adequate time for recuperation and growth between workouts. Proper application of the Power Factor Training system requires a maximum of no more than three workouts on three nonconsecutive days each week (such as Monday, Wednesday, and Friday), which further allows adequate time for full recovery and growth to occur. As your strength increases, that training frequency is reduced.

In fact, one of us (Sisco) was forced to take a six-week layoff after injuring his back (performing a full-range clean and press with 225 pounds). During that period, he also had the flu and was inactive. When he returned to the gym six weeks later, it was with the full intention of doing a very light workout, just to get used to training again. However, as soon as he started to train, he realized that the protracted off-time had filled his muscles with a recharged power—more power in fact than he had ever displayed! His overhead press weight went up to a phenomenal 510 pounds, while his bench press weight shot up to 600 pounds—a full 75 pounds past his previous best!

A similar, though less dramatic, increase occurred for John Little. He too was forced into a four-week period of relative inactivity. When he returned to the gym, his overhead press went up to 415 pounds for a triple (whereas before he couldn't even get 400 pounds off the pins), while his bench press went up to 540 pounds for a triple!

These results, along with the observations of Mike Mentzer and Michael Sherman and the clinical studies of exercise physiologists, reveal not only that trainees need a lot less time in the gym than had been universally believed (particularly by the periodization or cycling advocates), but that peak overload on a progressive basis performed over a given unit of time is the sole factor responsible for muscle growth. Strategically predetermining certain months in which to reduce your muscular overload and perform higher reps alternated with periods of moderate intensity with moderate reps, or any other such reduction in muscular output, is an absolute waste of time as far as stimulating increases in size and strength are concerned. Knowing these facts regarding the requirements for muscle growth, there is absolutely no excuse for the serious bodybuilder or powerlifter to train with less than all-out effort each and every workout.

As described earlier, periodization got its start when Soviet bloc Olympic coaches began the use of steroids for their athletes. The human body cannot withstand the massive doses of the drugs on a continual basis, so training intensity was reduced during the periods of no drug use and increased during periods of heavy drug use. This cycling of intensity was erroneously taken as the reason for the great strength increases. The truth is that it was the drugs that had to be cycled, not the training intensity.

COMPARING INDIVIDUALS

Q: Can I compare my Power Factor and Power Index to someone else's?

A: The simple answer to this question is no. There are many reasons, a few of which deserve some elaboration. Many bodybuilders and strength athletes refuse to believe that size and strength are related. To support this erroneous contention, they invariably point to two individuals and note that one of them is smaller and less massive than the other, yet the smaller individual can lift more weight. A contradiction? Only an apparent one.

What they've failed to consider in their example is the fact that accurate comparisons between individuals such as this cannot be made, as there are just too many independent variables to consider. It may very well be true that the smaller individual has a sixteen-inch arm and can curl 150 pounds, while the larger one has a seventeen-inch arm and can curl "only" 135 pounds. However, the individual with the sixteen-inch arm will be even stronger when his arm has grown to seventeen inches, because that size increase will be due to increased muscle strength. Likewise, the bigger individual will be even stronger when his arm measures nineteen inches. In some instances, the variance in strength can be due to leverage differences; the smaller arm may have shorter bones so that it lifts the weight a shorter distance, thereby providing the smaller individual with a decided advantage in demonstrating strength.

Another contributing factor could be the existence of favorable attachment points. For example, if one individual's biceps tendon is attached closer to the elbow joint, he will have a pronounced leverage advantage. Other factors influencing strength development include neuromuscular efficiency. A cubic inch of one individual's muscle may be capable of producing more power than a comparable amount of another individual's.

Because of these and other differences among individuals, meaningful comparisons are difficult to make. Comparisons are best made only by the individual measuring himself over a given period of time. The Power Factor and Power Index are intended to be used only as a relative indicator of whether or not your muscular overload and corresponding strength are increasing.

POWER FACTOR TRAINING'S EFFECTIVENESS

Q: Why is Power Factor Training more effective than other forms of training?
A: Power Factor Training is the most effective training method simply because it delivers the highest overload to the muscles. Further, this system takes into account the physiologic principles of recovery and growth after this superior form of overload has been applied. When these two aspects of training have been followed, the net gain is always progressive and superior results.

Knowing this, it further stands to reason that the most productive training method for a person to utilize in his quest for optimum strength and muscle size is that of Power Factor Training. This doesn't mean that all other training methods are bad, nor that unless you use Power Factor Training you're doomed to failure. Conventional training methods deliver some results, to be sure, because they do provide some form of overload to the muscles. However, they don't provide maximum overload to the muscles and a precise, mathematical method of gauging both muscular output and progress. Only Power Factor Training provides these.

BODYBUILDING APPLICATIONS

Q: I'm a bodybuilder, and I like to lift heavy weights. What difference will developing strong ligament strength in addition to muscle strength have on my physique?

A: To get the most out of your Power Factor Training, you should never neglect the exercises that build up the strength of the connective tissue and that accustom the body to the handling of extremely heavy poundages. The only way to obtain this power is through handling the heaviest possible poundages over short ranges of muscle action and, obviously, through the utilization of exercises that work the largest muscle groups of the body such as the thighs, the back, shoulders, chest, and arms.

In addition to increasing overall strength and mass and toning up the muscles and connective tissue, a Power Factor Training program increases confidence and enthusiasm. Handling extremely heavy poundages creates a positive mental outlook and sense of achievement. The poundages you used in ordinary movements and that seemed so heavy will appear as light as a feather after your Power Factor Training routine (should you decide to return to conventional training, that is!).

THE GENES OF A CHAMPION

Q: If I engage in Power Factor Training, will I become a champion bodybuilder?

A: There are many factors to consider when answering this question, not the least of which is genetics. As an example, no one would dispute the fact that being tall certainly would influence your chances of being a successful professional basketball player (Spud Webb notwithstanding) nor that the exact opposite would be true for someone who wanted to be a professional jockey. However, it's obvious that bouncing a basketball or running up and down a court won't have any effect upon your height, nor will riding a horse all day long make you a shorter individual. Your height in both of these cases is determined by your genetics.

Genetics—in particular, the genetic potential to develop inordinately large muscles—also plays a role in the success or failure of champion bodybuilders. Two of the most important factors in determining a muscle's size potential are the length of a given muscle (measured between the tendon attachments on each end) and the fiber density of the muscle itself. The longer the muscle, the greater the cross-sectional area when contracted, and thus the greater volume that muscle has the potential to reach.

Power Factor Training will help you realize all of your genetic potential. If you have extremely long muscle bellies throughout your entire physique, and if you also have the mental discipline, Power Factor Training could well make you a champion.

YOU'RE NEVER TOO OLD TO TRAIN

Q: I'm very interested in increasing my power and muscle mass. However, I'm over fifty years of age and believe I am too old to benefit from your system. Is there another activity that you can recommend for old-timers like me?
A: While we can empathize with concerns, we cannot at all agree that age is a barrier to engaging in Power Factor Training. In fact, a University of Southern California study involving a group of seventy-year-old men showed

significant improvement in muscular strength after an eight-week strength-training program. This underscores the fact that you're never too old to start strength training.

Remember that bigger muscles are stronger muscles, and stronger muscles contribute to any movement activity, improve posture, elevate your metabolism (which allows you to burn bodyfat more efficiently), and help to prevent injuries. Stronger muscles also mean more stable joints, which, as we get older, are usually the first areas to lose support and suffer pain.

With all these benefits in mind, we're inclined to recommend Power Factor Training. Not only are your joints, muscles, and connective tissue strengthened by proper Power Factor Training, but it produces benefits much more efficiently than does, say, walking or swimming, in a third of the time. Regardless of your age, if you can move a limb even a couple of inches, then you can move it against resistance and stimulate your muscles to grow stronger. However, be sure your physician gives you the OK before you participate in any vigorous exercise program.

STRENGTH VS. SPEED

Q: Even though I believe the principle that a stronger athlete is a better athlete, I'm not sure that a stronger athlete is a faster athlete. I need speed in my sport (martial arts). Will Power Factor Training be able to deliver it?
A: Absolutely! A stronger athlete is a faster athlete precisely because of the increased strength factor. Look at it this way. Let's say you want to press a 100-pound barbell overhead as fast as possible. If your deltoids, traps, and triceps muscles are capable of combining to press 102 pounds, then your speed of movement with

100 pounds will obviously be very slow. It might even take 5 or 6 seconds to move the weight to the locked out position. On the other hand, if the involved muscles are capable of pressing 200 pounds, you'll be able to press the 100-pound barbell in half a second and, in all probability, even less time. If your pressing ability is 250 pounds, then your speed of movement will be even more rapid. As skill is not significantly involved in pressing a barbell, the increase in speed is obviously due to the strengthening of the muscles.

If all else is equal, the stronger individual will also move the fastest, because he will have the greatest ratio of muscle mass to bodyweight. After all, if you add more horsepower to the engine of an automobile, it will move faster.

REALISTIC EXPECTATIONS

Q: How much muscle mass can you expect to build in one year of Power Factor Training?

A: It's been said that, if you are lucky enough to gain 10 pounds of muscle in one year, then you can consider yourself most fortunate. However, in light of the results we've been seeing in Power Factor Training, that belief may now be obsolete. For example, in one week of Power Factor Training, John Little gained 15 pounds after having remained at a bodyweight of 180 pounds for over 10 years. One might be tempted to say that he probably ate more during that week and trained less; therefore he gained 15 pounds of fat. However, he didn't alter his diet in any way. His waist size remained the same, while his Power Factor and Power Index all went up dramatically, which indicated a pronounced increase in strength. A stronger muscle is a bigger muscle, and a bigger muscle is a denser, heavier muscle. So the only reason for the increase had to be the adaptive bodily response (muscular overcompensation) to the superior overload imposed by his Power Factor Training. It's interesting to note that Little put on an additional 10 pounds over the next four weeks (twelve workouts) as his Power Factor and Power Index increased on a per workout basis.

For the majority of trainees, who still cling to other, less intense methods of training, 10 pounds a year may be a more realistic expectation, at least during the first few years. If you think 10 pounds per year isn't much (especially in light of the high-set, seven-day-per-week training methods most bodybuilders employ), then just imagine how little it actually is when measured on a day-to-day basis: 0.027 pound, or less than half an ounce. That's not even enough to register on a bodyweight scale!

With Power Factor Training, the trainees make palpable, measurable progress on a consistent basis. As evidenced by Little's success, it's not uncommon to gain upwards of 25 pounds, and many have used Power Factor Training to put on 40 or more pounds of muscle.

TRAINING FOR DEFINITION

Q: I want to put on muscle size as quickly as possible without putting on any fat in the process. In fact, I'd like to lose a bit of bodyfat too. How do I train for size and definition at the same time?

A: First off, you can't train for definition. Most people, when referring to definition training, mean long, arduous hours of low-intensity work, which does not build size but rather endurance or cardiovascular efficiency. To build size, you must do just the opposite, which means that training must be intense, infrequent, and relatively brief.

One of the basic concepts of exercise physiology is specificity, which means that your body will adapt to achieve only one of these goals but not both. We all possess what stress physiologist Hans Selye referred to as adaptation energy, and this adaptation energy must be spent 100 percent for building either size/strength or endurance. As a result, it would appear that you could more efficiently achieve your double-edged objective if, rather than divide this energy between the two, you instead trained specifically for size and simply reduced your caloric intake in the pursuit of definition.

PLATEAUS AND RECOVERY

Q: I was making good progress, but lately I haven't seen any gains. What's the problem?
A: This is one of the most asked questions in bodybuilding. To answer, we'll relate the true story of a man named Stanley. One of us (Sisco) received a telephone call from Stanley, in Massachusetts, who had been making good progress with his training but had recently hit a plateau that he just couldn't get past. Stanley is one of those guys with a tough-minded discipline that I can only admire. Despite his lack of progress in the gym, he did not get discouraged. He trained three days a week and never missed a workout. That's not easy. Most of us get demoralized when we give so much effort in the gym and see nothing for our exertion. Not to mention the fact that it's very tough to drag yourself to the gym and perform a decent workout when it feels as though every fiber of your body is saying, "Stop! I can't do it today."

Stanley and I did not have to talk very long before I realized that he had classic symptoms of overtraining. He lacked energy, he didn't feel like training, and he had not made the slightest progress in many weeks. I explained to him that this is the pit into which everyone falls as they get stronger. As your muscles become more powerful, they can perform workouts that really tax the rest of the body's organs like the liver, pancreas, and kidneys. Those organs don't grow along with the muscles, so as you get stronger, you have to cut back on training frequency.

I told Stanley to take three weeks off of all training. He said there was no way he could stay out of the gym that long. Actually, this is a common problem with serious bodybuilders. Mike Mentzer runs into the same resistance when he counsels brief and infrequent workouts. Psychologically, when you want to make progress, it is very difficult to do what seems like nothing. It feels like throwing in the towel or admitting defeat in some way. But the truth is that your body needs time to recover. Time off is not wasted time; it's time that is critical to the growth process. It took a lot of talk to convince Stanley but, to his credit, he took three weeks off of all training.

Two months later he called me back with results that surprised both of us. His strength had increased in every area of his body, and his shrug power had skyrocketed. His first workout after the layoff was a personal best. Now he's training once every nine days! (Before he was training four times in nine days. That's eighteen days between workouts for the same body parts.) The table shows the numbers he sent me in a letter. Stanley did not include his times for lifting, so I don't know his Power Factor or Power Index numbers. Still, his total shrug weight went from 15,300 pounds to 25,280 pounds after doing nothing for three weeks. When was the last time you had such a productive three-week period?

Think about that. Three weeks of no training, no supplements, no "light weight, high reps," nothing but sitting on his ass for three weeks. And his progress outpaced everybody's.

His training buddies couldn't believe their eyes. There's Stanley, who found it "very tough" to do 20 reps with 400 pounds now hoisting 505 pounds for 16 after

---

HOW STANLEY BENEFITED FROM LESS FREQUENT TRAINING

■ **OCTOBER 11**

365 lb.	20 reps
400 lb.	20 reps (very tough)

Took 3 weeks off.

■ **NOVEMBER 8**

405 lb.	20 reps (easy)
455 lb.	20 reps
505 lb.	16 reps

Trained once every 9 days.

■ **DECEMBER 17**

405 lb.	20 reps
505 lb.	20 reps
600 lb.	12 reps

---

doing 455 pounds for 20! Next time back in the gym, he's playing with 600 pounds. And, as far as his buddies are concerned, he's "missed" the last twenty workouts!

SIZE GAINS VS. STRENGTH GAINS

Q: I seem to be able to increase my strength on a consistent basis, but I'm not seeing size increases of the same magnitude. Why?

A: We hope no one reading this thinks there is a difference between training for size and training for strength. The fact is, muscle size and strength are directly related. For a muscle to be stronger, it has to get bigger. And vice versa.

Gym lore like "Positives for strength and negatives for mass" is crap. If this were true, it would be possible to train with a negatives-only routine and develop huge muscle mass but no strength. Picture a guy with a twenty-inch bulging arm who can't bench 150 pounds. Likewise, a positives-only routine would yield huge strength from scrawny arms. Picture a 650-pound bench with a twelve-inch arm; not likely. But even though there is a direct relationship between muscle size and strength, one of the most common complaints of bodybuilders is that they are making progress as far as strength goes, but there is little or no increase in size or mass. Perhaps this dilemma is what gives rise to myths like needing different training for mass than for strength.

The strength of a muscle fiber, like the strength of a steel cable, is proportional to its cross-sectional area. In basic terms, if a given muscle is to be twice as strong, it has to have twice the cross-sectional area. But to understand exactly what that means in terms of muscle measurements, you need to do a little work with geometry. I know some bodybuilders hate this mathematical stuff, but it's the key to learning the truth about what's going on with your training and inside your muscles.

Suppose you have a muscle in your body that is 3 inches in diameter. The top circle in the figure represents a muscle of that size. This muscle has a cross-sectional area of 7.07 square inches, according to the formula for area of a circle (πr^2, where π is 3.14159 and r is the muscle's radius). Suppose that you train hard in the gym for a period of time and increase your strength by a very respectable 50 percent. Let's say you go from benching 240 pounds for 10 reps to benching 360 pounds for 10 reps. Pretty good progress for a seasoned lifter. For the associated muscle to increase its strength by that 50 percent, it must increase its cross-sectional area by 50 percent. So its new area is one and a half times 7.07, or 10.61 square inches.

The bottom circle in the figure represents a muscle with the area of 10.61 inches. But when you measure it, the increase in size will seem to be less. Why? Because people don't usually measure the area; they measure the

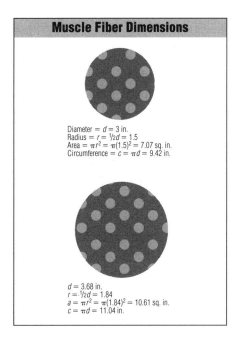

Muscle Fiber Dimensions

Diameter = d = 3 in.
Radius = r = $\frac{1}{2}d$ = 1.5
Area = πr^2 = $\pi(1.5)^2$ = 7.07 sq. in.
Circumference = c = πd = 9.42 in.

d = 3.68 in.
r = $\frac{1}{2}d$ = 1.84
a = πr^2 = $\pi(1.84)^2$ = 10.61 sq. in.
c = πd = 11.04 in.

circumference, or distance around. As you can see from the figure, the circumference increases much less than the area. So your muscle strength will always increase faster than the circumference of your muscle; it's a law of geometry.

Furthermore, a muscle is actually made up of millions of individual muscle fibers bundled together. If your muscles contained surplus intramuscular fat (fat contained in the muscle itself), it could be burned off as a result of your exercise, and the muscle fibers could expand into the area previously occupied by fat. Result: zero change in muscle size. In fact you could lose the more plentiful subcutaneous fat that most of us have too much of, and the muscle could expand itself into that area. Lose an inch of fat off your arm at the same time you pack on an inch of triceps size, and you net out at zero increase in arm size on the tape measure.

Also, your arm or leg or whatever is not 100 percent muscle. Bone, fat, ligaments, tendons, blood vessels, skin, and other components take up space. These components don't grow with exercise, so even though your muscle increased its area 50 percent through training, you'll see less change in the size of an entire leg that contains all that other stuff. If that's not enough, 60 percent of a muscle is water, so if you are a little dehydrated when you take your measurements, you won't see all the increase you could.

These factors together conspire to make size gains a lot harder to achieve than strength gains. But that doesn't change the fact that to get one, you need the other. Just be glad strength gains are so easy to measure with meaningful precision. That's what will keep you on the road of steady progress.

POWER FACTOR TRAINING AND THE CHAMPIONS

Q: You say Power Factor Training is the most efficient training system, but the guys up on the Olympia stage, the top guys in the sport, say they don't use your system. Why not?

A: There are several reasons, but perhaps the biggest is that the guys on the Olympia stage don't care about efficiency in training. Every top bodybuilder since the days of Larry Scott uses a maximum-volume approach to weight training. They perform workouts up to twice per day, six days per week. Routines such as these involve 20 to 30 sets of exercise per body part and workouts of three to four hours in duration. They are, quite literally, the most inefficient systems in use.

And the dirty little secret of the Olympia-caliber bodybuilders is that they spend between $20,000 and $50,000 per year in the black market to obtain about two dozen different drugs.[1] These drugs are illegal to obtain without a prescription, and some of them cannot be obtained in the United States even with a prescription. (Getting caught with them carries the same penalties as getting caught with heroin or cocaine.) These drugs greatly improve the body's ability to recover from the stress of exercise and to respond to the slightest stimulation. A person who is loaded up with all these drugs could do nothing but paddle a canoe and develop a massive upper body. And that's the problem. Once a person's body chemistry is so radically enhanced, all bets are off as to what elements of his training are working best.

As for the rest of us, we can't afford to overtrain with mega-volume routines because we simply won't be able to make progress without the same (dangerous) drugs. We need a training system that gives us the best results with a minimum of training. The Power Factor and Power Index are a means to exactly measure whether or not your training is giving you maximum gains for minimum effort. That's what efficiency means.

Remember, pro bodybuilders aren't even looking for efficiency. They try to get absolute maximum gains by using absolute maximum effort. They are looking at performing as many sets as possible as frequently as possible, even if it means performing thousands of useless sets or hundreds of useless workouts in a year. Even if it means using massive chemical help. Even if they die trying. And some do.

ANGLE TRAINING

Q: Are multiple exercises really necessary in order to attack the muscle from different angles?
A: This piece of misinformation is getting passed around so much it is becoming institutionalized. Is there a school

of certification for personal trainers that does not teach this as fact? Let's take a look at one of the most basic examples of this hypothesis at work: wide-grip barbell curls to attack (don't you love the term *attack*?—sounds as if General Patton devised the plan) the "inner biceps" and narrow-grip barbell curls to attack the "outer biceps."

In fact, the biceps muscles operate the elbow joint, which is just a simple hinge. There is nothing exotic happening at the elbow joint; it just bends up and down. Further, as with all muscles, the places where the muscle connects to the bone don't change. So every time the muscle is contracted, it pulls between the same two points of connection, moving the forearm upward while bending the elbow joint. That is all it can ever do.

Knowing that, how can a wide grip or narrow grip on a bar affect the operation of the direction of contraction of the muscles or the direction of travel of the elbow joint? It can't. The muscles are going to contract in a straight line between point A and point B in all cases. However, by operating the elbow joint with forces that are not in line with the direction of travel, you will introduce lateral shear forces to the joint. For example, picture a fence gate that swings on two hinges. The direction of travel in which those hinges are made to operate is forward and backward to open and close the gate. But suppose a 200-pound man sits on top of the gate, introducing a downward shear force. Now when you operate the gate, there is extra stress on the hinge because it has to support a force generated from an angle it was not designed to hold. The result is either a broken hinge or extra wear and tear, eventually leaving it damaged.

The same is true for your elbow joint. It is designed to work in an up-and-down motion, so side-to-side forces are not good for it. They impede its operation, and that is exactly why I think this particular bit of gym lore came into being. It's harder to do, so it must put more focus on just one part of a muscle to the exclusion of another part, right? I doubt it.

Try, for example, to do a one-handed dumbbell curl (caution: use a very light weight) by placing your hand behind your back then operating your elbow in a normal curl fashion. It's very difficult. There is no way you could perform that exercise with the same weight that you use in a standard curl. Does the fact that you are forced to use a lighter weight make that exercise superior? No, it makes it inferior. The multiple shear forces placed on the joint and tendon connections force the muscles to perform support functions that reduce their power to operate the hinge joint. The name of the game is maximum muscular overload, under optimal conditions, for any given muscle or group of muscles.

So why does virtually everyone counsel hammer curls, concentration curls, wide grip, narrow grip, cheat curls, cable curls, seated curls, standing curls, lying curls, incline curls, ad nauseam? What is the difference in the operation of the hinge joint and the connection points of the muscles? There isn't any. What's best? The one that, for you, generates the highest intensity of muscular overload—the highest Power Factor and/or Power Index.

Having said all of that, there is still a small dilemma. There are over six hundred muscles in the body and some pretty complex muscle groups like those in the back. Some muscle groups work simultaneously through compound angles and rotational directions. What needs to be done is a proper research study of various isolation movements versus compound movements for major muscle groups. We already have some evidence that you can isolate certain muscles in a group, but are three or four separate exercises in any way better than one compound exercise? And what specific exercises yield the highest intensity for the greatest number of people? Until a proper scientific study is conducted, all you can do is experiment with the exercises you think are working for you by measuring the intensity they generate. But ten different exercises for biceps? Forget it.

AEROBICS AND ANAEROBICS

Q: I don't want to ignore my cardiovascular fitness, but will those workouts affect my recovery ability? And will the high impact of running be detrimental to muscle building because of the jarring effect?

A: We get a lot of questions about aerobics as it relates to affecting recovery from strength training. If strength training were the only thing that a person were doing, it would be ideal to do absolutely nothing between workouts so as to allow maximal recovery. But not only is that impractical, it's also narrow-minded. Strength training is only one of three parts of fitness, the others being cardiovascular endurance and flexibility.

After a productive workout (one that stimulates new muscle growth), the body's first priority is to fully recover from the stress of the exercise. After it has recovered, it will grow any extra muscle that it requires. Most people's concern is that performing any aerobics between weight-lifting workouts will slow down the recovery process. It probably does, but if the aerobics is low intensity, which it should be, it shouldn't make much demand on the body's anaerobic system, so the effect will be negligible. It's a worthwhile trade-off, as cardiovascular fitness is critical to good health. If you are keeping proper track of your intensity numbers, you will spot the effects of too much aerobic exercise by seeing a decline in your strength progress. That's what happens to guys whose "aerobic" workout consists of donning a forty-pound backpack and running hills.

Damage from jarring is a very important point. Part of the recovery process includes repairing any bone, tendon, ligament, muscle, or other damage done during an exercise. It is logical for your body not to increase its biceps strength when the tendon has started to tear off the bone. The first priority should be to repair the tendon. So it's not the jarring itself that can cause problems, it's the damage caused by too much jarring that can slow down recovery and therefore slow down growth. What's too much? Well, a ten-year-old can jump off the roof of a house without causing too much jarring to his body, but an eighty-year-old can miss his step at a curb and break a hip.

FINDING YOUR SWEET SPOT

Q: When finding your sweet spot, is it just trial and error? Do you just add a few reps here and a few reps there?

A: There exists a great deal of physiological variation between individuals. Among the variations that can affect lifting weights are the length of bones, the insertion point of the muscles along the bones, the ratio of fiber types that muscles are made of, the efficiency of the neural muscular pathway, the ability to process ATP, the speed of cellular waste removal, and many others. For this reason, two people who seem to have approximately the same amount of strength (for example, they can both perform 3 reps with 300 pounds), can actually have peak muscular output occur under different set and rep schemes. One of them might be able to generate a maximum Power Factor of 2,200 pounds per minute by performing 3 sets of 20 reps with 225 pounds, while the other person is able to generate his maximum intensity of 2,600 pounds per minute with 4 sets of 14 reps with 260 pounds. If either of them followed the other's set/rep/weight scheme, he would generate less than the maximum intensity of which he is capable. He would be off his sweet spot.

Once you understand this concept, you realize how arbitrary an edict like "3 sets of 10 for six months" really is. Finding the optimum combination of sets/reps/weight is a process of experimentation with trial and error. Training to failure on at least one set will serve as a valuable guide. For instance, suppose you perform 2 sets of 20 reps then perform a third set to failure with the same weight and end up doing 37 reps. It's an indication that you might have started with too low a weight or too few reps in the first place. Next time out, try increasing the weight on the first two sets and/or increasing the reps. If this yields you a higher Power Factor and/or Power Index, you are heading in the right direction. By the way, if every workout is productive (and it should be!), your sweet spot will move around a bit because you are a different, stronger man (or woman) every time you come back to the gym.

Worried that you might not have hit the absolute high point of your spot? Don't. It's a logical impossibility to be certain that you hit your best on any given day. (That goes for you, Carl Lewis and Albert Einstein.) But remember this: If your intensity numbers are going up, you are absolutely, positively making progress.

REST TIME

Q: Your routines don't stipulate exact rest times between sets or between exercises. Why not?
A: Because you can judge that better than we can. Specifying a fifteen-second rest between sets might be

perfect for a twenty-year-old who plays water polo, but it will be too short for a sixty-five-year-old who plays shuffleboard. Rest time is one of four variables (the others being, weight, sets, and reps) that you can adjust in order to generate the highest intensity of overload. Just be mindful that while you are resting, your muscular output is zero pounds per minute, and that gets averaged into your total numbers.

If you give yourself too little rest, your next set (or exercise) will be less than the maximum of which you are capable. If you take too long a rest, your average output will be less than maximal. Don't be afraid to experiment a bit.

THREE SEPARATE WORKOUTS

Q: I find the leg workout (leg presses and toe presses) very demanding. I think I could make better progress if I left those exercises for a third, separate workout. Is that OK?
A: It's not only OK, it's the kind of experimentation that everyone should be prepared to do. The sole arbiter of whether or not to make any adjustment in your training regimen is whether or not doing so will increase your ability to maximize muscular output. Nothing else is relevant.

ORDER OF EXERCISES AND EXERCISE SUBSTITUTIONS

Q: I find it hard to do barbell shrugs right after standing barbell presses. Is it OK to change the order of exercises? Also, I think I do better with decline bench presses than flat bench. Is it OK to make that substitution?
A: These questions fall into the same category as the previous one. There is nothing sacrosanct about the order of exercises in Power Factor Training, or in any other

training program for that matter. The sequence of exercises should never be made to conform to edict or to unproven hypotheses regarding overload. The only element of variation that is important is this: Will the change I am going to make enable me to overload the muscle group in question to a greater degree? That answer will be evident in your Power Factor and Power Index numbers.

The same is true for substituting exercises. We discovered, through trial and error, which compound movements deliver the most muscular overload for most people. But there is great variation among individuals. If you are a person who discovers, through measurement and comparison, that you get higher triceps numbers from weighted dips than from close-grip bench presses, then do what gives you the higher numbers. Any other answer would be bodybuilding dogma instead of objective rationality.

MIXED PROGRESS

Q: On my last workout, four of my exercises showed improvement, but one actually declined. How can that be, and what should I do?

A: This is normal. Muscle recovery is both localized and systemic, so it is possible for you to make gains in all areas except one or two. There is also variation in the composition of the muscles in the same individual, so it would be unreasonable to expect all muscle to progress at an identical pace. Your analysis shows that you have a lagging body part or two that cannot progress as fast as the rest of your muscles.

When this happens, try leaving that exercise off your next workout (which is actually two workouts away, as you are always alternating between Workouts A and B) in order to allow additional rest time for that muscle group. However, if three out of five of your exercises suddenly do not show improvement, it is time to adjust your training frequency by adding one extra day of rest between all workouts. If you again fail to show improvement in three or more exercises, then add yet another day of rest into your training frequency.

Don't worry about losing what you have gained. All the data we have collected suggests that it takes several weeks to lose a measurable amount of strength. It is far more likely that your time off will be more productive than any time you might spend in the gym.

NOTE

1. Drug free or die, *Ironman*, 111 (November 1996); Drugs vs. Natural—the future of bodybuilding, *Muscular Development*, 134 (February 1996).

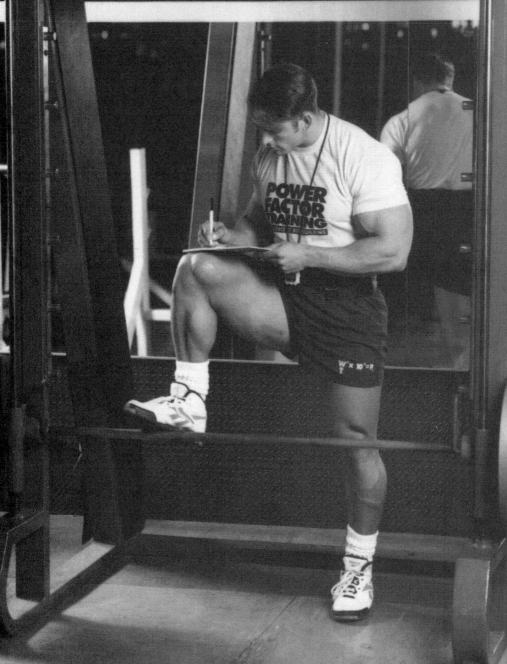

14

Your Logbook

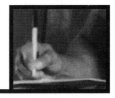

This section contains blank forms that you are authorized to photocopy for your personal use only. These forms make up a critical and indispensable component of Power Factor Training. They provide the means to numerically analyze every exercise and workout and to graph your progress or lack thereof. If you don't use these forms, you will simply overtrain blindly with strong-range partials in place of overtraining blindly with conventional exercises and methods.

The information in your logbook will enable you to determine what techniques work best for you.

THE WORKOUT RECORD FORM

Every time you perform a workout, you will use the Workout Record form. It allows you to record the weight, reps, sets, and time for each exercise, as well as the total time taken for your entire workout. The information on this sheet can be used to tell the whole story of whether your individual exercises

WORKOUT RECORD

Date: ____ / ____ / ____

Start Time: _____   Finish Time: _____   Total Time: _____

■ Exercise:

Weight Reps Sets	Weight Reps Sets	Weight Reps Sets	Weight Reps Sets	Weight Reps Sets	Weight Reps Sets
× ×	× ×	× ×	× ×	× ×	× ×
Subtotal = lb.	Subtotal = lb.	Subtotal = lb.	Subtotal = lb.	Subtotal = lb.	Subtotal = lb.

Exercise 1:   *Total Weight _____ lb.   Time: _____ min.   Power Factor _____ lb./min.   Power Index _____*

■ Exercise:

Weight Reps Sets	Weight Reps Sets	Weight Reps Sets	Weight Reps Sets	Weight Reps Sets	Weight Reps Sets
× ×	× ×	× ×	× ×	× ×	× ×
Subtotal = lb.	Subtotal = lb.	Subtotal = lb.	Subtotal = lb.	Subtotal = lb.	Subtotal = lb.

Exercise 2:   *Total Weight _____ lb.   Time: _____ min.   Power Factor _____ lb./min.   Power Index _____*

■ Exercise:

Weight Reps Sets	Weight Reps Sets	Weight Reps Sets	Weight Reps Sets	Weight Reps Sets	Weight Reps Sets
× ×	× ×	× ×	× ×	× ×	× ×
Subtotal = lb.	Subtotal = lb.	Subtotal = lb.	Subtotal = lb.	Subtotal = lb.	Subtotal = lb.

Exercise 3:   *Total Weight _____ lb.   Time: _____ min.   Power Factor _____ lb./min.   Power Index _____*

■ Exercise:

Weight Reps Sets	Weight Reps Sets	Weight Reps Sets	Weight Reps Sets	Weight Reps Sets	Weight Reps Sets
× ×	× ×	× ×	× ×	× ×	× ×
Subtotal = lb.	Subtotal = lb.	Subtotal = lb.	Subtotal = lb.	Subtotal = lb.	Subtotal = lb.

Exercise 4:   *Total Weight _____ lb.   Time: _____ min.   Power Factor _____ lb./min.   Power Index _____*

■ Exercise:

Weight Reps Sets	Weight Reps Sets	Weight Reps Sets	Weight Reps Sets	Weight Reps Sets	Weight Reps Sets
× ×	× ×	× ×	× ×	× ×	× ×
Subtotal = lb.	Subtotal = lb.	Subtotal = lb.	Subtotal = lb.	Subtotal = lb.	Subtotal = lb.

Exercise 5:   *Total Weight _____ lb.   Time: _____ min.   Power Factor _____ lb./min.   Power Index _____*

OVERALL WORKOUT: *Total Weight _____ lb.   Time: _____ min.   Power Factor _____ lb./min.   Power Index _____*

Exercise Subtotal = Weight × Reps × Sets ■ *Power Factor = lb./min.* ■ *Power Index = Total Weight × Power Factor ÷ 1,000,000* showed progress and were productive or were unproductive. Filling in these forms represents your advancement to the realm of a higher-technology, rational, scientific strength training.

THE EXERCISE/WORKOUT PERFORMANCE RECORD FORM

To show the progress of each exercise and of Workouts A and B, use the Exercise/Workout Performance Record form. At a glance you will be able to see your progress measured in the total weight you lifted and the associated Power Factor and Power Index numbers. Use a separate page for each exercise and for Workout A and Workout B.

GRAPHS

The graphs are used to display the information in the Exercise/Workout Performance Forms. By graphing your Power Factor and Power Index, you'll be able to see at a glance the rate of progress you are achieving. Also, plateaus and declines due to overtraining (or improper training) will be impossible to ignore. These graphs will provide all the evidence that you, or any skeptic in the gym, will need to verify your tangible, objectively measured progress.

Note that the Power Factor number is plotted on the left y-axis (vertical axis) and the Power Index number is plotted on the right y-axis. Note also that the Power Index scale is logarithmic.

EXERCISE/WORKOUT PERFORMANCE RECORD

■ Exercise:

Date	Total Weight	% Change	Power Factor	% Change	Power Index	+ or − Change

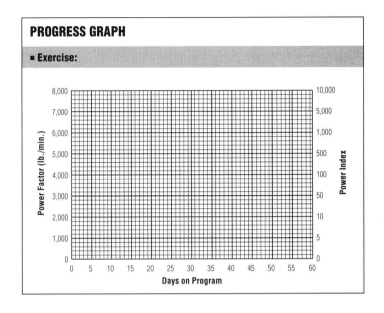

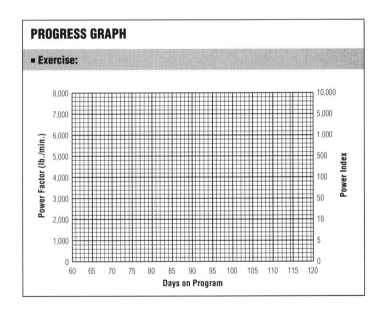

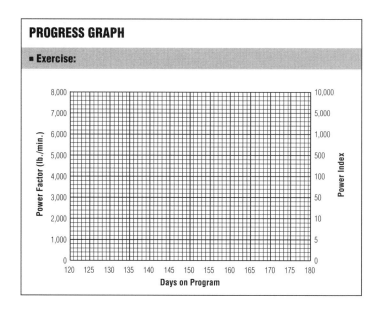

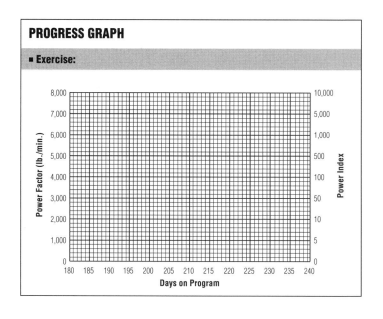

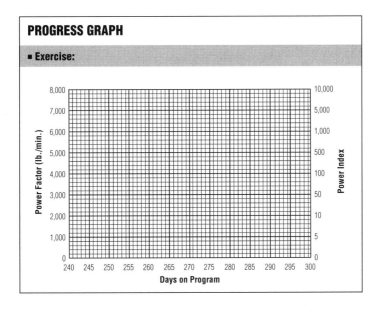

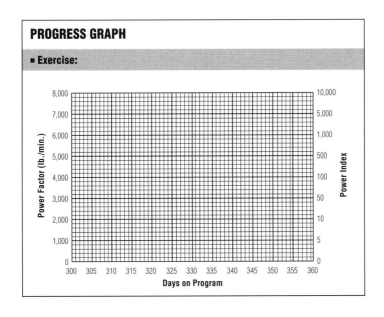

Resources

ACCESSORIES

Over the years we have discovered some really useful accessories that will enable you to get much more out of your Power Factor Training workouts.

Lifting Hooks
During exercises like lat pulldowns, barbell shrugs, and dead lifts, the amount of time that you are able to keep going is often limited by the strength in your hands and fingers. This is unfortunate, as those muscles are comparatively weak. Lifting hooks are a tremendous help in this area. They distribute the weight over your entire hand and wrist and enable you to continue to overload your larger muscles long after your grip would have let go. Hooks work much better than lifting straps for most people, because they require no finesse or technique in getting uniformity of grip in both hands. They are highly recommended.

Hooks are available in a one-size-fits-all version that is suitable for supporting weights up to about 300 pounds

($19.95 + $4.95 shipping and handling). There is also a super-heavy-duty version that can support weights up to the limits of human capacity ($29.95 + $4.95 shipping and handling). To order the heavy-duty hooks, provide a measurement of wrist circumference.

Crunch Strap

Conventional crunches are a great exercise for the abdominal muscles, but they don't allow you to add intensity as the muscles get stronger. This limitation is overcome with the use of a clever device called the crunch strap ($29.95 + $4.95 shipping and handling). The crunch strap is designed to attach to the low pulley of a weight stack so that weight can be added to the exercise. Once the added intensity of weight is incorporated into this exercise, your abs can develop to their maximum capability.

Lifting Belt

Nearly every exercise in Power Factor Training can be performed more safely with a good-quality weight belt. We would never perform a standing barbell press, squat, or dead lift without wearing a belt. We found an excellent-quality all-purpose belt suitable for all but the most advanced lifters. It features a large six-inch width and a hook and loop fastener. It's very comfortable and requires no breaking in. Specify size: S-M-L-XL ($29.95 + $4.95 shipping and handling).

Gloves/Wrist Wraps

We've found the best lifting gloves in the world. Period. These gloves are made by the Harbinger Company and have TechGel inserted into panels inside the glove for extra comfort and grip enhancement. They also have a CoolMax lining to keep your hands cool, dry, and comfortable by transporting moisture away from the skin. Best of all, they incorporate a patented leather wrist wrap that securely supports your wrist during exercises like standing barbell presses, bench presses, barbell curls, and others. We've tried scores of gloves over the years, and these are the only way to go. They are indispensable for all pressing movements. Specify size: S-M-L ($29.95 + $4.95 shipping and handling).

Software
We are developing a Windows 95™ Power Factor Training software program. This software will automate all logbook and graphing functions, automatically preengineer workouts of progressive overload, create progress reports, and more. Release date is summer 1997.

How to Order
These products are available by mailing to Power Factor, 10400 Overland Road, Suite 383, Boise, ID 83709 or by calling (800) 376-6117 with your Visa or MasterCard. Please note that the phone operators take orders only and cannot answer your training-related questions.

How to Contact the Authors
You can reach us via
- our Web page (http://www.precisiontraining.com)
- e-mail (Sisco@precisiontraining.com)
        (Little@precisiontraining.com)
- or regular mail to the address given for placing orders.

Train smart!
PETE SISCO AND JOHN LITTLE